Cybelle F. Barreto Medeiros Linard
Andrelina N. Coelhode Souza
Josenilda M. Cavalcanti

Antinociceptive effect of eugenol

Cybelle F. Barreto Medeiros Linard
Andrelina N. Coelhode Souza
Josenilda M. Cavalcanti

Antinociceptive effect of eugenol

in mice

ScienciaScripts

Imprint

Any brand names and product names mentioned in this book are subject to trademark, brand or patent protection and are trademarks or registered trademarks of their respective holders. The use of brand names, product names, common names, trade names, product descriptions etc. even without a particular marking in this work is in no way to be construed to mean that such names may be regarded as unrestricted in respect of trademark and brand protection legislation and could thus be used by anyone.

Cover image: www.ingimage.com

This book is a translation from the original published under ISBN 978-3-330-75761-5.

Publisher:
Sciencia Scripts
is a trademark of
Dodo Books Indian Ocean Ltd. and OmniScriptum S.R.L publishing group

120 High Road, East Finchley, London, N2 9ED, United Kingdom
Str. Armeneasca 28/1, office 1, Chisinau MD-2012, Republic of Moldova, Europe
Printed at: see last page
ISBN: 978-620-8-29160-0

SUMMARY

"Never confuse knowledge with wisdom.

One helps you to earn a living, the other to build a life."

S. Carey

To God for allowing me to do this work;

To my parents, Raul de Abreu Medeiros and Maria Erileide Façanha Barreto Medeiros, for their lifelong dedication to my studies;

To my husband Roberto Sérgio Sobreira Linard for the moments of absence he understood, for his contribution, for his revisions, but above all for his affection, companionship and encouragement in all the difficult moments of this journey; To my daughters Jûlia Teresa Medeiros Linard and Laura Teresa Medeiros Linard for their companionship, love and joy.

To my brothers, Raul Jr., Rômulo and Régis, for their affection and encouragement, which was essential for me to complete this journey.

ACKNOWLEDGMENTS

To the animals whose lives were taken for the sake of science.

Professor Andrelina Noronha Coelho de Souza for accepting to be my supervisor and for guiding this work;

To the members of the examining board (Professor Henrique Leal Cardoso, Professor Pergentino José da Cunha Sousa), for accepting the invitation, for their analysis and collaboration on this work;

To the teaching staff of the Academic Master's course;

To the Postgraduate Program in Physiological Sciences;

To Jô Malveira, more than a companion on this journey, for her encouragement, friendship, dedication and help in carrying out the experiments, which was essential for the completion of this work;

My friend Danùbia for her cheerfulness, company and help in carrying out the experiments;

To my uncle Erivan Façanha, who contributed to the development of this work;

To Cristiane Calado for her technical support, friendship, scientific and personal guidance;

To Karol Oliveira and Roney Feitosa for their friendship, companionship and collaboration in carrying out the experiments. To my friends Glaydson and Renata for their help in the final stages;

To my colleague Ariclécio Oliveira for his technical support, availability, attention and guidance, all of which were important in carrying out this work;

To Natàlia Celedônio, Rômulo Porto, Valéria Leonhardt, Anna Patricia, Renalison Pereira, Magna Marinho for their friendship;

To my friends Alana Pires and Sabrina Fontenelle for their companionship and words of encouragement;

To the employees Ecila and Lindalva, always with a smile on their faces, for their availability, attention and information, which only made the Master's course easier;

To Mauro, Franck, Gleidson, Bento and Pedro;

To the funding bodies and collaborators FUNCAP, UFC and Faculdades Christus;

To all those who, although not mentioned, helped in some way so that this work could be completed.

SUMMARY

Eugenol is a phenolic derivative, chemically known as 4-allyl-2-methoxy-phenol, commonly known as clove essence, as it is present in large quantities in the essential oil of clove (*Eugenia aromatica*), but is also present in cinnamon, sassafras and myrrh. It has various pharmacological effects, including antimicrobial, anti-inflammatory, spasmolytic, antiseptic, antipyretic, antioxidant and antinociceptive. The aim of this study was to investigate the local anesthetic effect of eugenol administered intraplantarly in mice and to compare it with the effect of capsaicin and lidocaine. To this end, we investigated the effect of eugenol, capsaicin and lidocaine in the formalin test. Eugenol at doses of 0.01, 0.1, 0.3, 1, 3 and 10µg/sitio, administered intraplantarly, did not increase nociception compared to the control in the first phase of the test. In the formalin test, eugenol reduced nociception by 70.69%, 43.71%, 53.76%, 54.98% and 64.57% respectively at doses of 0.1, 0.3, 1; 3 and 10µg/sitio, proving most effective at a dose of 0.1 µg/sitio, suggesting its effect on pain of neurogenic origin, which corroborates the results presented in the literature where eugenol, at low concentrations, is a reversible inhibitor of nerve activity. Pre-treatment with capsazepine and the destruction of afferent C fibers confirmed the action of eugenol on TRPV1 receptors, since eugenol did not reduce the nociception caused by formalin in either test. Capsaicin, compared to the control, was effective in reducing the nociception generated by formalin at doses of 0.01, 0.1, 0.3, 1, 3 and 10µg/sitio in the first phase of the test. This effect is probably due to the inhibition of voltage-dependent calcium channels by both capsaicin and eugenol. Lidocaine was used as a positive control in the test at doses of 0.01, 0.1, 0.3, 1, 3 and 10µg/sitio. Its effect proved effective in reducing the nociception caused by formalin in the neurogenic phase of the test, at all the doses tested. However, the anesthetic effect of eugenol at a dose of 0.1 µg/sitio was greater than that of lidocaine at the same dose. This effect is probably due to the action of eugenol and lidocaine on voltage-activated sodium channels, which are important for the initiation and propagation of action potentials in excitable cells, including sensory neurons. We can therefore conclude that eugenol in small doses does not increase nociception; it has a local antinociceptive effect, probably due to its inhibitory action on TRPV receptors[1] ; eugenol, capsaicin and lidocaine have a local antinociceptive effect in the first phase of the formalin test.

KEY WORDS:

Anesthetics; Eugenol; Pain measurement; Lidocaine

1 INTRODUCTION

Medicinal plants are of great importance in the treatment and cure of various ailments, mainly through the use of their essential oils. Their study in order to clarify their constituents, biological activities and adverse effects is important for scientific proof of their effects. Low costs and accessibility are factors that favor the research and use of natural products.

Eugenol, which is present in several essential oils, has attracted the interest of scientists due to its fat-solubility, low toxicity and biological activities.

Its proven biological activities include: antimicrobial (ESCOBAR, 2002); anti-inflammatory (KIM, et al, 2003); spasmolytic; antiseptic; antipyretic (FENG & LIPTON, 1987); antioxidant (STOHS et al, 1986; MANSUY et al, 1986; TAIRA et al, 1992; NAGABABU & LAKSHMAIAH, 1994; ABRAHAM, 2001); prevents anaphylactic reaction (KIM et al, 1997).

It is also used in the composition of clove-based perfumes, as a flavoring for non-alcoholic drinks, chewing gums, sweets, ice cream, chocolates, bakery products, jellies, puddings and tobacco, as well as a raw material for obtaining vanilla (KIM et al, 2003; COSTA, 2000, KOTHARI et al, 2004, RAGHAVENRA et al, 2006). In the fight against pain, it has analgesic and local anesthetic activity (ESCOBAR, 2002; DALLMEIR & CARLINI, 1981; SIEMONEIT et al, 1966).

Pain can be defined, according to the Taxonomy Committee of the International Association for the Study of Pain (I.A.S.P.), as an unpleasant sensation and experience associated with actual or potential tissue damage or described as such damage (MERSKEY & BOGDUK, 1994; MILLAN, 1999). It can be classified according to the type of damage and/or the mediators involved as: nociceptive, neurogenic, neuropathic and psychogenic, which are associated, respectively, with excessive stimulation of nociceptors, damage to neural tissue, dysfunction of a nerve or psychological factors (MILLAN, 1999). The discovery of low-toxicity, low-cost products that have anti-inflammatory, analgesic and anesthetic effects is promising for advances in the treatment of pain.

Local anesthetics are weak bases, mostly esters or amides, which act on the axon, reversibly blocking the generation and conduction of the nerve impulse. These drugs act on any part of the nervous system (ROCHA et al, 2002). Eugenol has been used in fish farming as an anesthetic and is important for reducing the hyper-motility of fish, which is a considerable source of injuries during handling and/or transportation procedures (INOUE et al, 2003; VIDAL et al, 2006).

1.1 ESSENTIAL OILS

Essential oils are volatile oily liquids extracted from various parts of plants (roots, stems, bark, leaves, flowers, inflorescences, seeds) using specific processes. They often have a pleasant aroma and are almost always biologically active. They are unstable when in contact with air, light, heat and humidity (MATOS, 1975).

Their chemical composition varies depending on genetic, physiological and environmental factors. In other words, in addition to the genetic determination of the plant, environmental conditions such as time of collection, season, soil constitution and climate can determine significant variations in the constitution of essential oils (SIMOES et al, 1999).

Essential oils are made up of ketones, hydrocarbons, alcohols, aldehydes, ethers, esters and phenols, among others, but a mixture of phenylpropanoid or terpenoid derivatives predominates (SIMOES et al, 1999).

1.2 EUGENOL

Eugenol is a phenylpropanoid derivative, chemically known as 4-allyl-2-methoxy-phenol or 2-methoxy-4-(2-propenyl-phenol) (MORRISON & BOYD, 1961), commonly known as clove essence (Figure 1), as it is present in large quantities in clove essential oil (*Eugenia aromàtica*) (ESCOBAR, 2002).

It is also present in the essential oils of various plants, including: *Ocimum tenuiflorum* (KOTHARI et al, 2004); *Caryphyllus aromaticus; Ocimum gratissimum*, widely used in Brazil to treat intestinal disorders and easily found in north-eastern Brazil (MADEIRA et al, 2005); *Eugenia caryophyllus, Dicipelium cariophyllatum, Pimenta dioica, Croton zehntneri* (KIM et al, 1997; UEDA-NAKANURA et al, 2006). It can also be found in nutmeg, cinnamon, bay leaves, sassafras, myrrh and others (KIM et al, 1997).

It is synthesized biologically from the amino acid phenylalanine via the phenylpropanoid metabolic pathway: shikinate, phenylalanine and unamic acid (SENANAYAKE, 1977).

It has a liquid and oily consistency, light yellow in color, with a characteristic aroma and a burning, spicy taste (ALMEIDA, 2004). Its melting and boiling points are -9 and + 253^0 C (BUDAVARI, 1996). When in prolonged contact with air, it is unstable, becoming more viscous and dark reddish in color.

It can be obtained by fractionating the essential oils of plants, extracted from different parts of them (leaves, flower buds, fruit, thin branches), using water vapor distillation (CRAVEIRO et al, 1981).

It has low solubility in water and is completely soluble in chloroform, ethyl alcohol, fat and ether. As it is lipophilic, it is rapidly absorbed (ESCOBAR, 2002) and is able to penetrate biological membranes and reach intracellular targets such as mitochondria, where it inhibits the oxidation of NADH (reduced nicotinamide adenine dinucleotide), reducing ATP levels (USTA et al, 2002).

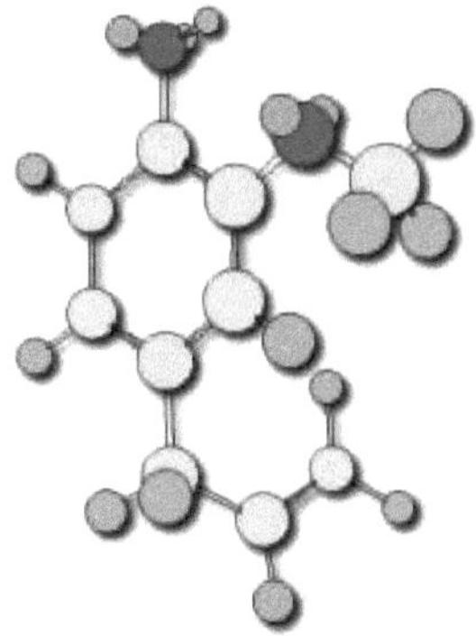

THREE-DIMENSIONAL STRUCTURE

FLAT STRUCTURE

Figure 1: Three-dimensional and flat structure of the Eugenol molecule

It has been used since the 15th century and was introduced into dentistry in 1873 to form zinc eugenolate together with zinc oxide and be applied directly to the dentin cavity (ESCOBAR, 2002).

The bond between eugenol and zinc oxide occurs due to a chelation reaction to form zinc eugenolate. Zinc eugenolate, when analyzed structurally, has the conformation of zinc oxide grains embedded in a zinc eugenolate matrix. When exposed to aqueous media such as saliva and dental fluid, the eugenolate hydrolyzes, releasing zinc hydroxide and eugenol, which diffuse from the dentin to the pulp, where they produce anti-inflammatory and anesthetic effects (MARKOWITZ et al, 1992).

Eugenol is also used in mouthwash and toothpaste formulations (ESCOBAR, 2002).

According to Leal-Cardoso (1994), in a study of frog skeletal muscle, eugenol (0.1-2.5 mM) blocked the contraction induced by 80mM K^+ , an effect attributed to a decrease in the release of Ca^{++} from intracellular stores. At higher concentrations of this compound (3-12mM), eugenol promoted contraction independent of extracellular Ca^{++} and blocked by procaine, suggesting that eugenol was releasing Ca^{++} from the sarcoplasmic reticulum.

1.2.1 Pharmacological properties

The biological effects of eugenol depend on its concentration and the time of exposure to the tissue (ESCOBAR, 2002).

It has several pharmacological properties, among which we can highlight: antimicrobial, anti-inflammatory, antioxidant, modulator of immune responses, anticarcinogenic, cardiovascular, antinociceptive and local anesthetic.

We can also highlight spasmolytic, antiseptic, muscle relaxant activity (ALMEIDA, 2004), reduction of tongue edema induced by plant poisoning (DIP et al, 2004), anthelmintic activity in ruminants (PESSOA et al, 2002), antipyretic (when administered peripherally or centrally, reducing fever by central action, like acetaminophen) (FENG & LIPTON, 1987).

1.2.1.1 Antimicrobial activity

The antimicrobial activity of eugenol has been attributed to its phenolic structure which, at higher concentrations, causes the degeneration of proteins in the cell membranes of bacteria, resulting in damage to the cell membrane. At lower concentrations, it tends to stabilize the cell membranes, preventing bacteria from penetrating the dental canal (MARKOWITZ et al, 1992), making it useful in the treatment of oral diseases caused by pathogenic microorganisms (ESCOBAR, 2002).

1.2.1.2 Anti-inflammatory activity

Eugenol suppresses the expression of cyclooxygenase 2 (COX-2) in mouse macrophages activated by lysophosphatidylcholine (LPC) (KIM et al, 2003) and inhibits the activity of lipooxygenase-5 in human polymorphonuclear cells (RAGHAVENRA et al, 2006), thus having an anti-inflammatory effect.

It modulates some immune responses, including an anti-inflammatory effect, but the mechanism of action has not yet been established.

Eugenol has the property of inhibiting platelet aggregation and thromboxane B_2 activity (SHARMA et al, 1994; NAIDU, 1995).

1.2.1.3 Antioxidant activity

The antioxidant activity of eugenol is determined by its methoxyphenolic structure which inhibits lipid peroxidation by scavenging reactive oxygen species intermediate radicals (STOHS et al, 1986; MANSUY et al, 1986; TAIRA et al, 1992; NAGABABU & LAKSHMAIAH, 1994; ABRAHAM, 2001).

Due to its antioxidant properties and antimicrobial activity, eugenol has been used as an important food preservative (STOHS et al, 1986; MANSUY et al, 1986; TAIRA et al, 1992; NAGABABU & LAKSHMAIAH, 1994; ABRAHAM, 2001).

It also has a modulating effect on intracellular concentrations of antioxidant substances such as glutathione and the enzyme glutathione-N-transferase (DRUKARCH et al, 1997; ROMPELBERG et al, 1996; BOUTHILLIER, CHARBONNEAU and BRODEUR, 1996; STOHS et al, 1986).

According to Ito et al (2005), eugenol also has antioxidant activity against the oxidation of LDL-cholesterol molecules due to its metal-reducing properties and the formation of inactive methyl-eugenol complexes that do not react with oxygen.

1.2.1.4 Activity in immune responses

In a study carried out by Kumaravelu (1996), eugenol reduced carbon tetrachloride-induced damage to red blood cells and inhibited mast cell degranulation both *in vitro* and *in vivo*, preventing anaphylactic reactions (KIM et al, 1997).

According to Sieben (2001), eugenol promotes an immune response mediated by T cells, but the molecular mechanism of action is still not completely clear. T helper cells are important in the immune response, which can be mediated by the production of cytokines. Interleukin-2 (IL-2) is a representative of the interleukins produced by the activation of T helper cells (preceding T cell proliferation) and also participates in the regulation of other immune cells, including B lymphocytes, macrophages and killer T cells (SMITH, 1988).

1.2.1.5 Anticarcinogenic activity

Some studies have attributed anticarcinogenic activity to eugenol (REDDY et al, 1993; REDDY, 1996, 1997; AL-HARBI et al, 1995) since eugenol suppressed the mutagenicity induced in *Salmonella typhimurium* TA100 by aflotoxin [B1] and N-methyl-Nnitro-N-nitrosiguanidine (FRANCIS et al, 1989) and in *Salmonella typhimurium* TA98 by dimethylbenzanthracene (AMONKAR et al, 1986).

It also reversibly inhibits glutathione-S-tranferase, thus indicating a protective effect against tumor growth and tumor resistance to drugs (ROMPELBERG et al, 1996). Due to its anticarcinogenic properties, it could be used as a cancer chemopreventive agent (KIM et al, 1997).

1.2.1.6 Effect of eugenol on the cardiovascular system

Eugenol, at concentrations of 10 to $1000\mu M$, promoted vasodilation of the artery pre-contracted by norepinephrine, by high concentrations of K^+ and by electrical stimulation, *in both in vivo and in vitro* experiments. These effects have been attributed to a blockade of calcium channels and inhibition of the contractile machinery (HUME, 1983; NISHIJIMA et al, 1999). Intravenous treatment of rats with eugenol induces arterial hypotension from a dose of 1mg/Kg in both anesthetized and awake rats. *In vitro*, eugenol showed vasodilator activity in a mesenteric bed precontracted by 60mM K^+ (LAHLOU et al, 2004).

1.2.1.7 Antinociceptive and anesthetic activity

Eugenol has antinociceptive, anti-inflammatory, analgesic and anesthetic activity.

Data obtained by Souza (2008) indicate that eugenol administered orally has a significant antinociceptive activity, which has been proven in three experimental models of nociception: the abdominal writhing test, the hot plate test and the formalin test.

The data obtained with the abdominal writhing test and the hot plate test indicate the action of eugenol on acute pain (BIGHETTI et al, 1999).

The anti-inflammatory properties of eugenol were detected through the inhibition of paw edema induced by carrageenan and dextran. It was also observed that eugenol reduced body temperature.

In low concentrations, eugenol inhibits nerve activity because it quickly penetrates the myelin sheath of a nerve fiber or bundle, blocking the generation and conduction of the nerve impulse and promoting an analgesic and local anesthetic effect (ESCOBAR, 2002; DALLMEIR and CARLINI, 1981; SIEMONEIT et al, 1966). The removal of eugenol from the site of action leads to a return to normality (ESCOBAR, 2002).

Anesthetic substances are often used to reduce the hyper-motility of fish, which is a considerable source of injuries during handling and/or transportation procedures (INOUE et al, 2003; VIDAL et al, 2006). Due to its anesthetic efficacy, low cost and lack of adverse effects, eugenol is a promising anesthetic for fish farming (SMALL, 2003).

Studies on the use of eugenol as an anesthetic in aquaculture arose from the need to find new effective, safe and low-cost substances (ROUBACH et al, 2005).

Vidal et al (2007) demonstrated that eugenol at a concentration of 50mg/L is efficient as a deep anesthetic, following the methodology proposed by Ross & Ross (1999), with regard to the induction and recovery times of anesthesia in the aquaculture of juvenile matrixâ fish. Increasing the concentrations of eugenol to 62.5, 75 and 100 mg/L only influenced the anesthetic induction time of the matrixâ juveniles. After anesthesia, recovery occurred regardless of the dose of eugenol.

The anesthetic effect of eugenol has already been demonstrated for various species of fish, among them: tambaqui, *Colossoma macropomum* (ROUBACH et al, 2005), pintado, *Pseudoplatystoma corruscans* (VIDAL et al, 2006), jundià, *Rhamdia quelen* (CUNHA et al, 2006) and sea bass, *Centropomus undecimalis* (SOUZA-JUNIOR and ALVES-JUNIOR, 2006), as well as eugenol's ability to reduce stress during transportation and handling (CUNHA et al, 2006).

1.2.1.8 Undesirable effects

Hume (1983) proved that eugenol, both *in vivo* and *in vitro*, has different types of toxicity and can cause the body: dermatitis, allergic reactions, liver dysfunction, disseminated intravascular coagulation and severe hypoglycemia. However, these effects are only observed at doses higher than 10^{-3} mol/L (ALMEIDA, 2004).

1.3 NOCIPATION

Nociception is the mechanism by which painful stimuli are transmitted to the central nervous system (FURST, 1999).

Nociceptive transmission is a mechanism that involves very complex interactions between peripheral and cerebral structures from the skin surface to the cerebral cortex (FURST, 1999).

The understanding of the mechanisms involved in the transmission of the pain process has progressed a lot in recent years, possibly due to the use of multiple experimental protocols, including behavioral studies, *in vitro* and *in vivo* electrophysiology, anatomical studies and mainly through molecular biology techniques (MILLAN, 1999, LEAL-CARDOSO et al, 2003).

Nooiocptive information is transmitted from the periphery to the central nervous system by two classes of primary afferent fibers whose cell bodies are located in the dorsal root horn:

♦ A delta fibers - myelinated fibers of small diameter, with a conduction velocity of 12 to 30m/s, conduct information of high incidence and low latency, responsible for the rapid or primary transmission of pain (FURST, 1999);

♦ C fibers - unmyelinated fibers, with a conduction velocity of between 0.5 and 2m/s, react to high intensity stimuli such as thermal, mechanical and chemical stimuli (FURST, 1999).

All tissues, with the exception of neutrophils in the central nervous system, are innervated by these afferent fibers. However, these fibers have different properties according to the tissue they innervate and can be classified into (MILLAN, 1999):

♦ Somatic afferents - innervate the skin, joints and muscles;

♦ Visceral afferents - innervate cardiovascular and respiratory tissues, the gastrointestinal tract, excretory and reproductive systems.

The primary afferent fibers make secondary synapses with numerous neurons in the superficial lamina of the dorsal root horn of the spinal cord, known as second-order neurons (LAWSON, 2002).

The second-order neurons cross the spinal cord to ascend to the spinothalamic tract, projecting their terminal fibers mainly to the thalamus. In the thalamus, the third-order neurons send axons through the internal capsule to the somatosensory cortex, where somatization of the nociceptive stimulus takes place, or send axons to the anterior cingulate gyrus, where the emotional component of pain is emitted (RUSSO & BROSE, 1998). This pathway is called the classic route, but there are other possible pathways involving different nerve structures (BESSON, 1999).

In addition, the spinothalamic tract seems to send axons to the midbrain and rostral pons, making synapses in nuclear complexes, including the raphe magnus nucleus (NMR). Both structures seem to be involved in the down-regulation of second-order neurons (MILLAN, 1999).

All the neurotransmitters involved in the descending inhibitory control of pain transmission, such as endogenous opioids, serotonin and noradrenaline, appear to inhibit the excitation of second-order neurons in the presence of noxious stimuli (RUSSO & BROSE, 1998; FURST, 1999; MILLAN, 1999).

There are several important sources where chemical mediators that participate in the perpetuation of the pain response are generated, including: injured and adjacent tissues, the vascular system, immune cells, sympathetic and sensory nerves, among others. In addition, there are complex mechanisms by which a transmitter can act via multiple receptors that are widely distributed throughout the peripheral or central tissues (MILLAN, 1999).

1.3.1 Nociceptive research

Nociceptive investigation can be carried out using various tests, including the abdominal writhing test, the hot plate test and the formalin test.

♦ The abdominal writhing test allows us to detect analgesics that act mainly peripherally, but can also detect those that act centrally, making it valuable for a comprehensive antinociceptive investigation (DERAEDT et al, 1980);

♦ The hot plate test is characterized by short-lived responses to high-intensity physical stimuli (GYIRES and TORMA, 1984). It is considered a sensitive test to analgesics that act at a central level. It can be used to evaluate and compare analgesic agents;

♦ The formalin test has a deep connection with tissue injury, which makes it a valid model of clinical pain. This test is useful not only for evaluating analgesic drugs, but also for elucidating pain and analgesia mechanisms. Formalin acts as a noxious agent and induces diffuse, moderate and long-lasting pain. It has also been postulated that peripheral pain mediated by formalin may be analogous to human post-operative pain (ABBOTT and FRANKLIN, 1986).

The painful experience begins in the nociceptor, a specialized primary afferent neuron, which responds to injury or the threat of injury to the body. The pain phenomenon initially involves transduction, sensitization and modulation of the painful stimulus. The mechanisms involved in transforming a damaging signal into a nerve signal, which make up transduction, were unknown for a long time and are now being better understood, especially after the discovery of the vanilloid receptor, which is responsible for transducing the stimulus.

1.4 CA CHANNELS^{++}

Calcium ion is essential for a wide variety of intracellular and extracellular processes in all organisms. Intracellularly, calcium is involved in the control of various cellular functions such as muscle contraction, hormone secretion and glycogen metabolism, as well as acting as a second messenger and enzyme co-factor. In the extracellular process, it participates in numerous essential functions, such as blood coagulation, cell adhesion, maintenance of skeletal integrity and regulation of extracellular excitability (BROWN, 1991).

The basal value of intracellular calcium, usually around 100 nM, is approximately 10,000 times lower than the concentration of extracellular ionized calcium, which is around 1 mM. Despite this favorable transmembrane electrochemical gradient, Ca is restricted in its entry into the cell and is mediated by specific channels and transporters in the plasma membrane.

Oscillations in the concentration of intracellular calcium are due to its exit from the cell through the membrane, but also to its mobilization from intracellular reserves.

This kinetics of calcium enables the activation of various metabolic processes (cardiac activity, transmission of signals to nerve cells, muscle contraction, among others) and the regulation of muscle and nerve functions.

Calcium channels can be classified as: voltage-dependent calcium channels and receptor-dependent channels. These two types of channels are functionally coupled, and there is interaction between them in the entry of calcium from the external to the intracellular environment (RASMUSSEN, 1993).

The flow of calcium through voltage-dependent channels is controlled by the electrical transmembrane potential, hence the name voltage-sensitive. According to their pharmacological and electrophysiological properties, six types of voltage-dependent calcium channels found in various tissues can be distinguished: L, N, P, Q, R and T.

L-type channels are activated by a strong depolarization which has little effect on their inactivation. They are located in skeletal muscle, cardiac muscle, smooth muscle, brain and retina. Their main role in muscle is the coupling of excitation and contraction by allowing extracellular calcium to enter the sarcoplasm.

The N, P, Q and R channels are also activated by strong depolarization. Inactivation of these channels, located in the presynaptic terminals, is slow. Their main role is the release of neurotransmitters. They couple action potentials to the release of neurotransmitters.

T-type voltage-dependent channels have a low conductance. They are activated by depolarization close to the resting potential. Their inactivation is rapid and reactivation requires strong hyperpolarization. They are located in the nervous system and in cardiac and vascular smooth muscle. Their main role is probably in the rhythmic action potentials of cardiac muscle cells and neurons.

1.4.1 Vanilloid receptors

The vanilloid receptor was discovered by Thresh (1946) and was so named because of its structural similarity to vanilla (NELSON, 1919). It is a 95 kDa transmembrane protein that belongs to the family of voltage-dependent receptors operated by calcium. They allow calcium to enter from the extracellular to the intracellular environment (CATERINA & JULIUS, 2001).

There are several types of vanilloid receptors $TRPV_1$, $TRPV_2$, $TRPV_3$ and $TRPV_4$, which are classified according to their specific activity (CATERINA, 2001; DAVIS et al, 2000).

They are polymodal, non-selective cation-binding channels expressed in nociceptors whose function is the chemical integration of pain and physical stimuli including heat and extracellular acidification (low pH) (SAITOH et al, 2007).

They can be activated by both chemical substances (such as capsaicin and lipid mediators) and physical agents (such as heat, low pH), promoting membrane depolarization due to the influx of sodium and calcium, i.e. opening selective cation channels (HARDIE et al, 1993; CATERINA et al, 1997; MONTELL et al, 1997).

Capsaicin, by activating TRPV receptors$_i$, promotes calcium influx, resulting in various intracellular events that lead to the release of neuropeptides from sensory neurons such as substance Pe and calcitonin gene-related peptide (CGRP) from peripheral and central terminals (GEPPETTI and TREVISANI, 2004). This influx of calcium can be inhibited by capsazepine, a TRPV1 receptor antagonist (CORRELL et al, 2004).

Eugenol acts on TRPV1 receptors, blocking them. This blockade inhibits pain transmission (YANG et al, 2003).

Eugenol promotes an inhibition of both voltage-activated sodium and calcium channels independent of TRPV1 receptors, and an inhibition of voltage-activated potassium (Kv) channels was also observed in trigeminal ganglion neurons and in heterologous systems using voltage clamp. This inhibition was observed in both capsaicin-sensitive and non-sensitive rat trigeminal ganglion neurons.

Pretreatment with capsazepine, which is known as a TRPV1 receptor antagonist, decreased the effect of eugenol on Kv, suggesting an involvement of TRPV1 receptors in the action of eugenol (LI et al, 2007).

As its pharmacological properties have evolved and become known, eugenol now has common, specific and selective uses, and has been used in different dental areas (ESCOBAR, 2002).

The great interest in studying it may be due to its many proven pharmacological effects and its low toxicity (LEAL-CARDOSO et al, 2002).

1.5 ANESTHETICS

Since the dawn of science, people have been looking for ways to eliminate pain. In March 1842, in Georgia, physician Crawford Williamson Long was the first to use anesthesia, using ether in an operative procedure.

The first local anesthetic used was cocaine, extracted from *Erythroxylon coca* leaves, isolated in 1860 by Albert Niemann.

Anesthetics are drugs used to reduce pain sensitivity. They can be subdivided into two classes: general and local anesthetics.

General anesthetics cause loss of sensitivity to pain with unconsciousness, amnesia, analgesia, muscle relaxation, abolition of reflexes and hypnosis. They can be administered by inhalation or intravenously.

Local anaesthetics are drugs used to reduce sensitivity to pain in localized areas of the body, without loss of consciousness.

Most anesthetic molecules consist of an aromatic part linked to a basic side chain by an ester or amide bond.

Anesthetics from the ester group are rarely used today, as they have a shorter action time and produce more allergic processes than those from the amide group. Examples of this group are: cocaine, procaine, benzocaine and tetracaine.

Anesthetics from the amide group are the most widely used today because they produce fewer side effects than those from the ester group. Examples of this group are lidocaine, mepivacaine and ropivacaine.

Anesthetic molecules are weak bases with a pKa value mainly in the 8-9 range, so that at physiological pH they are largely ionized, but not completely. Their common characteristics are a weak dipolar moment and hydrophobic hydration.

This way in which anesthetics group together in a closed space is the anesthetic phenomenon (YAMAMOTO et al, 2006). This is important in relation to their ability to penetrate nerve sheaths and axon membranes. The presence of an ester or amide bond is important due to metabolic susceptibility.

Ester-containing compounds are generally inactivated in plasma and tissues (especially the liver) by non-specific esterases. Amides are more stable and have a longer plasma half-life.

Anesthetics can act by two different mechanisms: unspecifically or based on the specific receptor theory. In the first mechanism, the action is on the membrane, affecting various membrane functions and not just sodium conductance, in a similar way to volatile anesthetics. The second mechanism proposes that local anesthetics act by directly binding to specific receptors in the sodium channel, blocking them.

Anesthetic potency is known to be temperature-dependent. For hydrophilic anesthetics this potency decreases and for hydrophobic anesthetics it increases as the temperature decreases (YAMAMOTO et al, 2006).

Another important factor concerns the type of procedure performed. Those that take place in the presence of an inflammatory process (such as drainage, apicectomies and endodontics) are more prone to anesthetic failure. There are two reasons for this. The first indicates that the anesthetic applied to a site with an altered pH would have less action due to the difficulty in dissociating the anesthetic salt (ROOD, 1977/1978). Another suggests that the greater vascularization of the inflamed site leads to faster absorption of the anaesthetic (HIDDING & KHOURY, 1991).

1.5.1 Potential for action

The nervous system, together with the endocrine system, enable the body to perceive variations in the environment (internal and external), to disseminate the changes that these variations produce and to carry out the appropriate responses so that homeostasis is maintained.

In the nervous system, neurons are the cells responsible for receiving and transmitting stimuli from the environment (internal and external). In order to carry out these functions, they have two fundamental properties: excitability and conductivity. Excitability is the ability of a cell to respond to stimuli. The response emitted by neurons resembles an electric current. Once excited by stimuli, neurons transmit this wave of excitation, called a nerve impulse, along their entire length at great speed and in a short space of time. This phenomenon is due to the property of conductivity.

The neuron's plasma membrane actively transports some ions, via channels, from the extracellular fluid into the intracellular medium and vice versa. This is how the sodium-potassium pump works, actively pumping sodium out, while potassium is actively pumped in. However, this pumping is not equitable: for every three sodium ions pumped into the extracellular fluid, only two potassium ions are pumped into the intracellular fluid. As the outflow of sodium is not accompanied by potassium in the same proportion, a difference in electrical charges is established between the intracellular and extracellular media - there is a deficit of positive charges inside the cell and the faces of the membrane remain electrically charged.

The electronegative potential created inside the nerve fiber due to selective permeability is called the resting potential of the membrane, with the outside of the membrane being positive and the inside negative. We then say that the membrane is polarized. When stimulated, a small region of the membrane becomes permeable to sodium (opening of sodium channels). The entry of sodium is accompanied by a small outflow of potassium. This whole process is called a depolarization wave. Nerve impulses or action potentials are caused by depolarization of the membrane beyond a threshold.

The action potential is a phenomenon by which a cell generates a depolarization or reversal of the membrane potential of the all-or-nothing type of short duration, being generated by the change in permeability to sodium ions (internally directed current) and potassium (externally directed current). This ionic current occurs through channels in the plasma membrane.

The channels are membrane proteins, all of which have a basic molecular structure, but their different ionic selectivity means that they have very different physiological functions. This selectivity is determined by the diameter, shape and nature of the electrical charges along the inner surface of the channel.

In general, there are two ways in which the function of the channels can be modified, either by blocking or by modifying the behavior of the gate. Either mechanism can cause an increase or decrease in excitability. The channels can also be selectively affected by different pharmacological classes. Sodium channels can be blocked by antiarrhythmic drugs, some anticonvulsants such as phenytoin and neurotoxins such as tetrodoxin and saxotoxin.

1.5.2 Na channels$^+$

Voltage-activated sodium channels play an essential role in initiating and propagating the action potential of neurons and excitable monocytes, cells of the endocrine system (HODGKIN and HUXLEY, 1952).

These channels have two "gates", one near the outer end of the channel, called the activation gate, and another near the inner end, called the inactivation gate.

Two types of channels are expressed in small neurons of the dorsal horn and trigeminal ganglion (NaV 1.8 and NaV 1.90) and play an essential role in the perception of pain (AKOPIAN et al, 1999). While a third type can be found in sensory neurons and neurons of the sympathetic nervous system (NaV 1.7) (LAURETTI, 2008).

In the axon, sodium channels are heterotrimeric proteins made up of protein subunits alpha (260,000 Da), beta 1 (36,000 Da) and beta 2 (33,000 Da). There are studies showing variants of the alpha protein subunit that forms the Na+ channel, which would have implications for altering the pain threshold in different tissues and between individuals

(OGATA and OHISHI, 2002).

Substances that interact with these channels reduce nociception. These include local anesthetics such as lidocaine (FERNANDES FRACETO et al, 2005) and eugenol (SOUZA, 2005; PARK et al, 2006).

Lidocaine, the reference drug for the study of new products with anaesthetic action, has a greater affinity for the open ion channel, the state generated during depolarization (FERNANDES FRACETO et al, 2005).

Other ion channels are expressed in the cytoplasmic membrane and are partly responsible for the difference between intra- and extracellular ion concentration. This is what happens with calcium ions. This difference is largely maintained by the low natural permeability of the cytoplasmic membrane to calcium (RASMUSSEN, 1993).

1.5.3 Local anesthetics

Local anesthetics are molecules that act mainly by blocking sodium channels, promoting the blocking of the inflow and propagation of action potentials, preventing the increase in voltage-dependent sodium conductance, causing loss of sensation without loss of consciousness.

In general, local anesthetics block conductance in small diameter nerve fibers more easily than in large diameter ones. However, the smallest fibers in peripheral nerves are the unmyelinated C fibers, and these are much less susceptible than the smaller myelinated A delta fibers. As nociceptive impulses are transmitted by A delta and C fibers, the sensation of pain is blocked more easily than other sensory modalities.

Amide-type local anesthetics have significantly improved the safety of anesthesia. They easily cross the blood-brain barrier, placenta and enter the circulatory system of the developing fetus. The primary site of biotransformation of local anesthetics is the liver (by microsomal mixed-function oxidases), with monoethylglycine and xylidide (potentially toxic) being the main biotransformation products.

The pH of an anesthetic solution and the pH of the tissue into which it is injected have a great influence on the nerve blocking action. Acidification of the tissue reduces the effectiveness of local anesthesia. Inadequate anesthesia occurs when local anesthetics are injected into an inflamed or infected area (MALAMED, 1993).

The undesirable effects of local anesthetics involve the central nervous and cardiovascular systems and are the main source of risk in the clinical use of local anesthetics.

Its main effect on the central nervous system is to cause stimulation. This produces restlessness and tremor with subjective effects ranging from mental confusion to extreme agitation. The tremor can evolve into actual convulsions and further increases in the dose produce central nervous system depression, with the main risk to life being respiratory depression.

The cardiovascular effects are myocardial depression and vasodilation. The decrease in myocardial contractility probably stems indirectly from the inhibition of sodium current in the heart muscle. The reduction in sodium intake leads to a decrease in sodium concentration, which in turn decreases intracellular calcium reserves and this reduces the force of contraction, mainly affecting the arterioles. Vasodilation is partly due to a direct effect on vascular smooth muscle and partly to inhibition of the sympathetic nervous system.

Local anesthetics associated with sympathomimetic vasoconstrictors, such as epinephrine and noradrenaline, can interact with non-selective beta blockers, MAO inhibitors and tricyclic antidepressants (HAAS, 2002).

The initial clinical signs and symptoms of central nervous system toxicity are of an excitatory nature, such as: difficult speech, chills, muscle contraction, tremors of the muscles of the face and distal extremities and symptoms of hot and flushed skin, generalized delirium, dizziness, visual disturbances such as inability to focus, auditory disturbances such as tinnitus, drowsiness and disorientation. Bilateral paresthesia of the tongue and perioral region is a sign of a toxic reaction due to the high levels of local anesthetic, but mild sedation or drowsiness may develop instead of excitatory signs. Excitement and sedation occur 5 to 10 minutes after the administration of a local anaesthetic and should serve as a warning of the possibility of a generalized tonic-clonic convulsive episode if plasma levels continue to rise.

For local pain relief, lidocaine, procaine and tetracaine are the most commonly used anesthetics.

1.5.4 Lidocaine

Lidocaine hydrochloride (2-diethylamino-2, 6-acetoxylidide hydrochloride) was the first amide-type anaesthetic to be synthesized and introduced into the clinic. It is resistant to hydrolysis and is still found today in different products. It has a pKa of 7.9 and a protein bond of 65%. Its onset of action is rapid (2 to 3 minutes) and it has a half-life of 90 minutes.

Local anesthetics such as lidocaine apparently block TRPV1 receptors by a mechanism that is still unclear. Lidocaine hydrochloride is currently used as a standard of comparison to verify the efficacy of other local anesthetics.

The maximum dose of lidocaine hydrochloride is 4.4 mg/Kg (not to exceed 300mg).

Drug interactions generally involve central nervous system depressants, such as narcotics, opioids, anxiolytics, phenothiazines, barbiturates and anti-histamines. When applied together, they potentiate the cardiorespiratory actions of local anesthetics.

In female mice, the intravenous LD_{50} of lidocaine hydrochloride is 21-31mg/kg and the subcutaneous LD_{50} is 203-304mg/kg, as shown in the drug leaflet for injectable lidocaine hydrochloride produced by Laboratòrio Probem - Laboratório de Produtos Farmacêuticos.

Today's local anesthetics act on any part of the nervous system and on any type of fiber, not just those that transmit pain, which causes temporary local paralysis.

The discovery of efficient local anesthetics, with specific action on the neurons that transmit pain, sparing the neurons responsible for muscle movement and touch, without potentially dangerous side effects and which do not cause the lethargic state that follows traditional anesthesia, is of paramount importance for the clinic (PATEL et al, 1993).

2. OBJECTIVES

2.1 GENERAL

To analyze the local anesthetic effect of eugenol administered intraplantarly in mice.

2.2 SPECIFIC

To investigate the local nociceptive effect of eugenol;

To evaluate the local antinociceptive effect of eugenol;

Elucidate the effect of eugenol on type 1 vanilloid receptors;

Compare the local effect of eugenol with the local effect of capsaicin and lidocaine.

3. MATERIALS AND METHODS

All the salts used were of analytical purity, and the experiments followed the ethical requirements of animal research.

3.1 MATERIALS

3.1.1 Experimental animals

In all the experiments, male *Swiss* mice weighing between 25 and 30g were used, from the Central Bioterium of the Federal University of Cearà and the Central Bioterium of the Christus College.

The animals were kept under controlled conditions of temperature (22 ± 2°C) and light (12-hour light/dark cycle) with free access to food and water before the experiments in the vivarium of the Higher Institute of Physiological Sciences, CCS, UECE.

At least three days before the experiments, the animals were transferred from the vivarium of the Higher Institute of Physiological Sciences, CCS, UECE to the Laboratory of Experimental Physiology (LAFIEX) of the same university, maintaining temperature and light conditions, grouped in a maximum number of 15 animals per box. The experiments were carried out in a quiet room, maintaining temperature control and always during the light phase of the cycle and in accordance with the guidelines for the care of laboratory animals and ethical considerations for investigations of experimental pain in conscious animals (ZIMMERMANN, 1983).

All the protocols used in this study were approved by the Committee for Ethics in the Use of Animals (CEUA) of the State University of Ceará, under opinion number 07199459-9 (11/06/2007).

3.1.2 Reagents, drugs and solutions

The following reagents, drugs and solutions were used:

♦ Capsaicin (Sigma Chemical, St. Louis, MO, USA);

♦ Capsazepine (Tocris Cookson, Baldwin, USA);

♦ Ethanol (Sigma Chemical, St. Louis, MO, USA);

♦ Eugenol (Sigma Chemical, St. Louis, MO, USA);

♦ Formalin (MERCK Laboratory, Darmstadt, Germany);

♦ Lidocaine (Laboratòrio de produtos farmacêuticos e Odontológicos S/A., Sp, Brazil);

♦ Sterile saline solution 0.9% (ADV, Ceará, Brazil);

♦ Tween 80 (Sigma Chemical, St. Louis, MO, USA)

Eugenol was prepared in a sterile saline solution containing 1% v/v Tween 80 followed by magnetic stirring.

The capsaicin solutions for intraplantar administration were prepared in a sterile saline solution of sodium chloride, 2% v/v ethanol, 1% v/v Tween 80 and then homogenized by magnetic stirring. The capsaicin solution used on the newborn animals to destroy the C-fiber was prepared as recommended by Holzer (1991), with 0.9% v/v sterile saline solution and 0.001% v/v Tween-80.

The capsazepine solution was prepared with a sterile saline solution of sodium chloride, 2% v/v ethanol, 10% v/v Tween 80, as described by Lee et al (2006).

The lidocaine solution was diluted in sterile sodium chloride saline from an ampoule bottle.

3.2 METHODS

3.2.1 Effect of intraplantar eugenol

Male *Swiss* mice were placed individually under an inverted glass funnel next to a mirror for an adaptation period of 20 minutes. After this period, $20\mu L$ of eugenol was injected into the left paw of each animal at doses of 0.01, 0.1, 0.3, 1, 3 and $10\mu g$/sitio. After injection, the animals were placed back under the glass funnel. The time the animal spent licking or biting its left paw was then timed, in the first five minutes and in the interval between fifteen and thirty minutes after the injection. This time is an indication of pain.

The control group consisted of animals that received $20\mu L$ of sterile saline solution containing 1% v/v Tween 80 in their left paw. In the control group, as in the experimental group, the animals underwent a period of adaptation.

At the end of the observation time for all the experimental procedures, the animals were sacrificed with a high dose of thiopental.

3.2.2 Formalin test

The pain test induced by intraplantar injection of formalin was used to evaluate the anesthetic effect of eugenol.

The animals were placed individually under an inverted transparent glass funnel next to a mirror to facilitate visualization for an adaptation period of at least 20 minutes.

After the adaptation period, the animals received a final volume of $20\mu L$ of the study compound in the left paw together with 2.5% formalin.(Figure 2, Figure 3, Figure 4) After intraplantar injection, they were placed back in the funnel for a period of 30 minutes. During this period, the time the animal spent licking or biting the paw where the formalin and eugenol or capsaicin or lidocaine was injected was timed, and this time was an indication of pain (HUNSKAAR et al, 1985, 1987; T0JELSEN et al, 1992).

The control group for the formalin test with eugenol consisted of animals that received a final volume of $20\mu L$ containing 2.5% formalin together with sterile saline solution with 1% v/v Tween 80 in the left paw. The control group for the capsaicin formalin test consisted of animals that received formalin in the left paw along with sterile saline solution of sodium chloride, 2% v/v ethanol, 1% v/v Tween 80, totaling a final volume of $20\mu L$. The control for the formalin test with lidocaine consisted of animals that received $20\mu L$ of 2.5% formalin and sterile saline solution in the left paw.

The tests were carried out at room temperature (22 ± 2°C) and in the absence of experimental factors that could affect peripheral blood flow, due to the high sensitivity of the response in the second (late) phase.

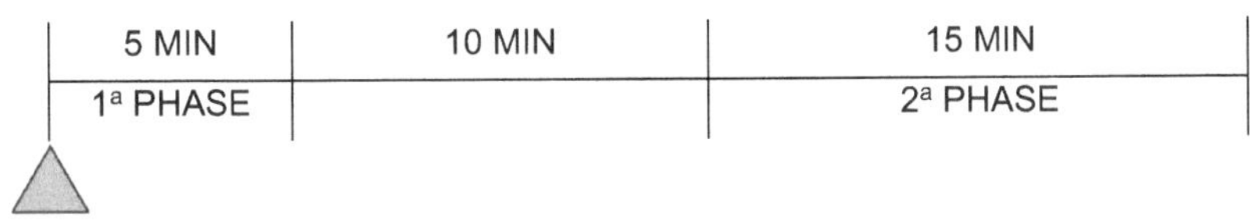

Figure 2: Formalin test with Eugenol

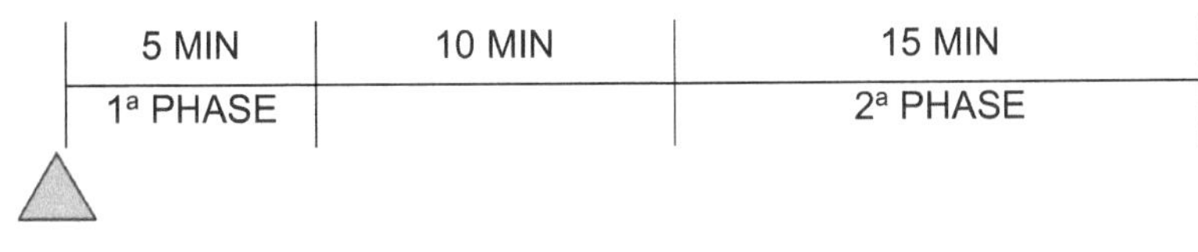

Figure 3: Formalin test with Capsaicin

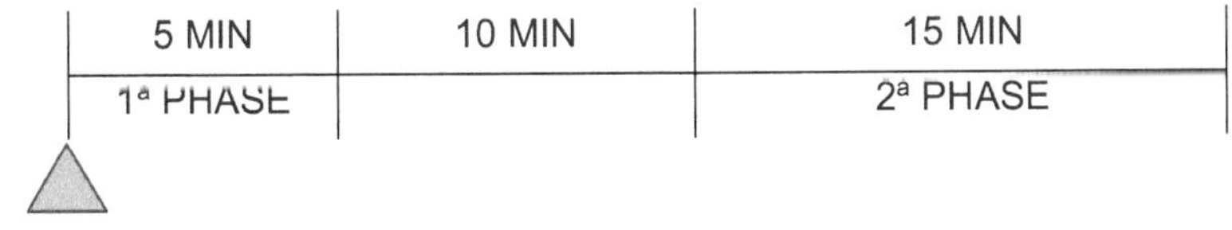

Figura 4: Formalin test with Lidocaine

3.2.3 Pre-treatment with capsazepine

The animals received an intraperitoneal injection of capsazepine at a concentration of 1mg/Kg, dissolved in 2% v/v ethanol, 10% v/v Tween 80 in a sterile 0.9% sodium chloride solution, 30 minutes before the experiment, in accordance with Joohyeng et al (2006). After this period, the formalin test was carried out together with eugenol at concentrations of 0.01, 0.1, 0.3, 1, 3 and 10 µg/sitio (Figure 5).

The control group received an intraperitoneal injection of capsazepine at a concentration of 1mg/Kg, just like the experimental group, 30 minutes before the experiment. After this period, the formalin test was carried out together with sterile saline solution containing 1%v/v Tween 80, totaling a final volume of 20µL.

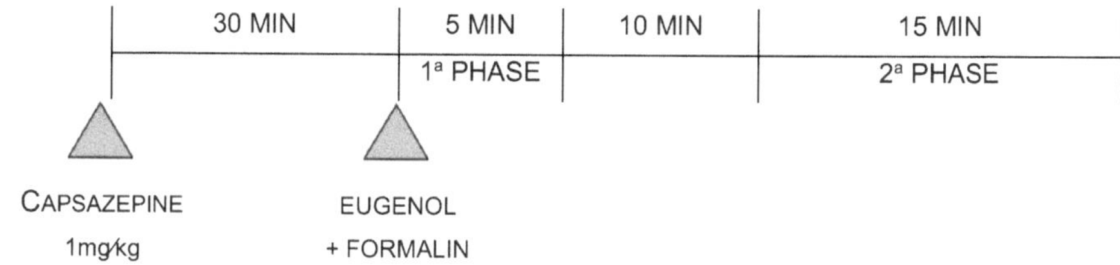

Figura 5: Formalin test with Eugenol in animals pre-treated with capsazepine

3.2.4 Participation of capsaicin-sensitive fibers

The animals were treated on the second day of life with capsaicin (50mg/Kg, 10µL) subcutaneously. After this treatment, the animals were used for six to seven weeks (BUCK and BURKS, 1983) in the formalin test together with intraplantar eugenol (Figure 6).

Before being used in the formalin test, the animals were subjected to the eye wipe test as described by Ikeda et al (2001). The aim of this test was to assess whether the degeneration of capsaicin-sensitive primary C fibers had actually occurred. Briefly, 20 µL of a 0.01% (w/v) capsaicin solution was instilled into one eye and the number of wiping movements that occurred in the subsequent one-minute period was counted. Animals that wiped their eyes a maximum of five times were considered to be desensitized. They were used three days after the eye cleaning test (Figure 6).

The control group consisted of animals that were given 10µL subcutaneously at birth of the vehicle used to dissolve capsaicin (saline solution and 0.001% v/v Tween-80). The eye cleaning test was carried out between six and seven weeks of age. Animals that wiped their eyes more than five times were considered non-desensitized and used in the formalin test together with eugenol.

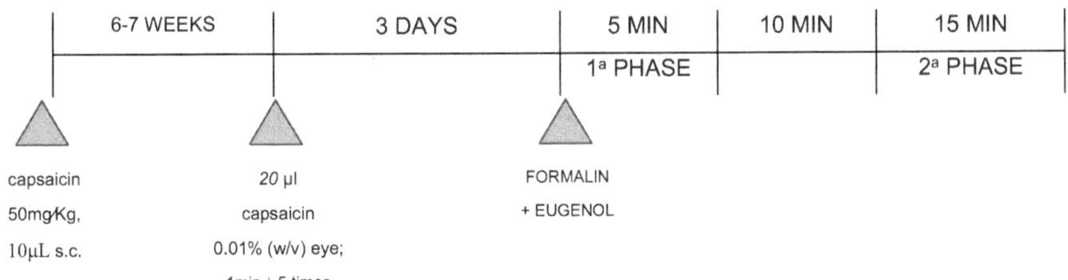

Figura 6: Formalin test with Eugenol on animals that had their C-fiber destroyed at birth

3.3 STATISTICAL ANALYSIS

The results are presented as the mean ± standard error of the mean (SEM), where n represents the number of animals.

The graphs shown here were created using SIGMA PLOT software.

Statistical significance was verified using SIGMA STAR software.

The results were statistically analyzed using the one-way ANOVA test compared to the control group. P values lower than 0.05 ($p \leq 0.05$) were considered to indicate significance.

4. RESULTS

In the graphical representations presented throughout this chapter, the ordinate axis represents the time in seconds spent by the animal licking its paw and the abscissa axis represents the control together with each of the doses tested.

The columns represent the average licking time and the data label, at the top of each column, the standard error of the mean (SEM). Gray columns represent the first phase of the test and red columns the second phase.

4.1. Evaluation of the nociceptive effect of eugenol.

When the effect of intraplantar eugenol was analyzed, in the first phase of the test, at doses of 0.01; 0.1; 0.3; 1; 3; 10µg/sitio it decreased nociception compared to the control. At a dose of 30 µg/sitio, eugenol increased nociception, but not significantly, in the first five minutes after injection compared to the control. However, at a dose of 100µg/sitio, eugenol increased nociception by $106.02 \pm 0.18\%$ (ANOVA, Kruskal-Wallis One Way Analysis of Variance on Ranks) compared to the control (Figure 7, Table 1).

[a]For the 2nd phase of the test, the increase in nociception was significantly observed at doses of 10, 30 and 100µg/sitio, respectively, at $46.40 \pm 0.21\%$, $86.40 \pm 0.61\%$ and $145.60 \pm 0.26\%$ compared to the control (ANOVA, Kruskal-Wallis One Way Analysis of Variance on Ranks) (Figure 7, Table 1).

4.2. Evaluation of the antinociceptive effect of eugenol administered intraplantarly in the formalin test.

Eugenol caused a reduction in formalin-induced nociception in the first phase of the test. It significantly (ANOVA, Dunnett's test) inhibited the response to painful stimuli at doses of 0.1, 0.3, 1, 3 and 10µg/sitio by $70.69 \pm 1.70\%$, $43.71 \pm 3.56\%$, $53.76 \pm 5.40\%$, $54.99 \pm 2.33\%$ and $64.57 \pm 3.51\%$, respectively (Figure 8, Table 2).

In the second phase of the formalin test, eugenol significantly reduced the nociceptive response (ANOVA, Dunnett's test) by $23.82 \pm 3.50\%$ at a dose of 0.1µg/sitio and at a dose of 0.01 µg/sitio it increased nociception by $10.78 \pm 4.14\%$ (Figure 8, Table 2).

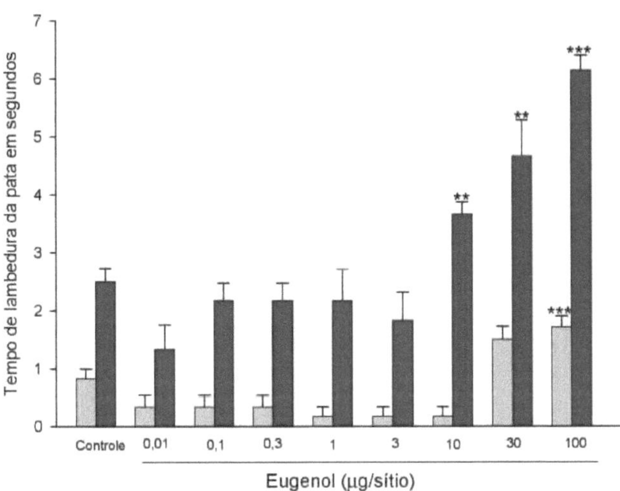

Figura 7 - Evaluation of the nociceptive effect of eugenol

(*) Statistically different from control **p < 0.05, compared to vehicle control (ANOVA, Tukey test); ***p < 0.05, compared to vehicle control (ANOVA, Dunn's test). The ordinate axis represents the time in seconds spent by the animal licking its paw and the abscissa represents the control together with each of the doses of eugenol tested. The columns represent the average licking time and the data label, at the top of each column, the standard error of the mean (SEM). n= 6 -7 animals. Gray columns represent the first phase of the test and red columns the second phase.

Treatment	Doses (µg/sitio)	Paw licking time (seconds) 1ª PHASE ⇑	% inhibition 1st PHASE	Paw licking time (seconds) 2nd PHASE ⇑	% inhibition 2nd PHASE
Control (vehicle)	-	0,83 ± 0,16	-	2,50 ± 0,22	-
Eugenol	0,01	0,33 ± 0,21	60,24	1,33 ± 0,42	46,80
	0,1	0,33 ± 0,21	60,24	2,16 ± 0,30	13,60
	0,3	0,33 ± 0,21	60,24	2,16 ± 0,30	13,60
	1	0,16 ± 0,16	80,72	2,16 ± 0,54	13,60
	3	0,16 ± 0,16	80,72	1,83 ± 0,47	26,80
	10	0,16 ± 0,16	80,72	3,66 ± 0,21**	146,40
	30	1,50 ± 0,22	180,72	4,66 ± 0,61**	186,40
	100	1,71 ± 0,18 ***	206,02	6,14 ± 0,26***	245,60

Table 1 - Evaluation of the nociceptive effect of eugenol 1st and 2nd phase of the formalin test

⇑ Values expressed as mean ± E.P.M.

**p < 0.05, compared to vehicle control (ANOVA, Tukey test);

***p < 0, 05, compared to vehicle control (ANOVA, Dunn's test)

% inhibition with values greater than 100 mean that the dose tested increased nociception in relation to the control

n = 6 - 7 animals

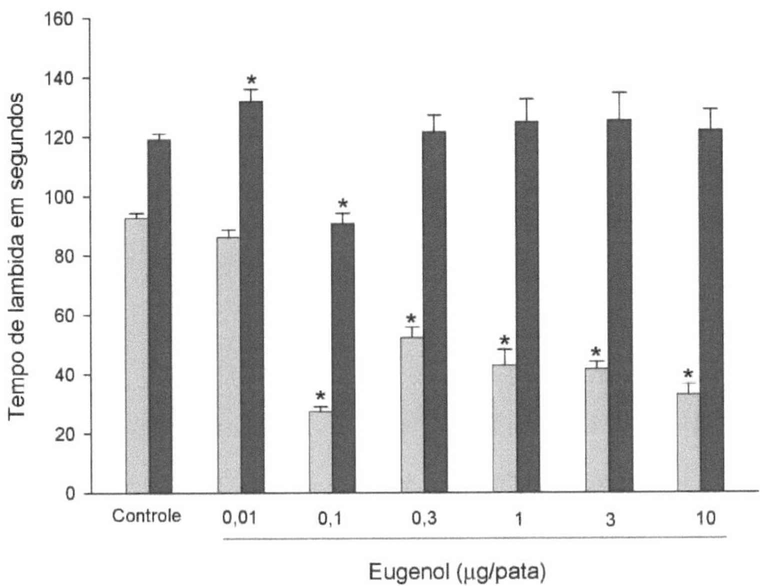

Figura 8 - Evaluation of the antinociceptive effect of eugenol, administered intraplantarly, in the formalin test

(*) Statistically different from the control *p< 0.05 (ANOVA, Dunnett's test). The ordinate axis represents the time in seconds spent by the animal licking its paw and the abscissa represents the control together with each of the tested doses of eugenol. The columns represent the average licking time and the data label, at the top of each column, the standard error of the mean (SEM). n= 6 - 7 animals. Gray columns represent the first phase of the test and red columns the second phase.

Treatment	Doses (µg/sitio)	Paw licking time (seconds) 1ª PHASE ⇑	% inhibition 1st PHASE	Paw licking time (seconds) 2nd PHASE ⇑	% inhibition 2a PHASE
Control (vehicle)	-	92,66 ±1.52	-	119,00 ± 2,04	-
Eugenol	0,01	86,16 ± 2,49	7,01	131,83 ± 4,14 *	110,78
	0,1	27,16 ± 1,70*	**70,69**	90,66 ± 3,50 *	**23,82**
	0,3	52,16 ± 3,56 *	43,71	121,50 ± 5,69	102,10
	1	42,85 ± 5,40 *	53,76	124,71 ± 7,72	104,80
	3	41,71 ± 2,33 *	54,99	125,42 ± 9,20	105,39
	10	32,83 ± 3,51 *	64,57	122,00 ± 6,96	102,52

Table 2 - Evaluation of the antinociceptive effect of eugenol administered intraplantarly 1ª and 2ª phase of the formalin test

⇑ Values expressed as Mean ± E.P.M.

*$p \leq 0.05$, compared to vehicle control (ANOVA, Dunnett's test)

% inhibition with values greater than 100 mean that the dose tested increased nociception compared to the control.

n = 6 - 7 animals.

4.3. Evaluation of the antinociceptive effect of eugenol in the formalin test in animals pretreated with capsazepine.

Pretreatment with capsazepine (1mg/Kg) reversed the antinociceptive effect of eugenol at doses of 0.1; 0.3; 1; 3; 10µg/sitio in the first and second phases of the formalin test (Figure 9, Table 3).

In the second phase of the test, the antinociceptive effect of eugenol was abolished at a dose of 0.1µg/sitio. However, at doses of 0.01 and 3µg/sitio, eugenol significantly increased nociception (ANOVA, Dunnett's test) by 33.81 ± 13.34% and 44.93 ± 6.90% respectively (Figure 9, Table 3).

4.4. Evaluation of the effect of eugenol in animals with destroyed C-fiber.

Eugenol at doses of 0.01, 0.1, 0.3, 1, 3 and 10µgZsitio administered intraplantar together with formalin in animals with destroyed C-fiber did not significantly (ANOVA) reduce nociception in the first or second phase of the formalin test (Figure 10, Table 4).

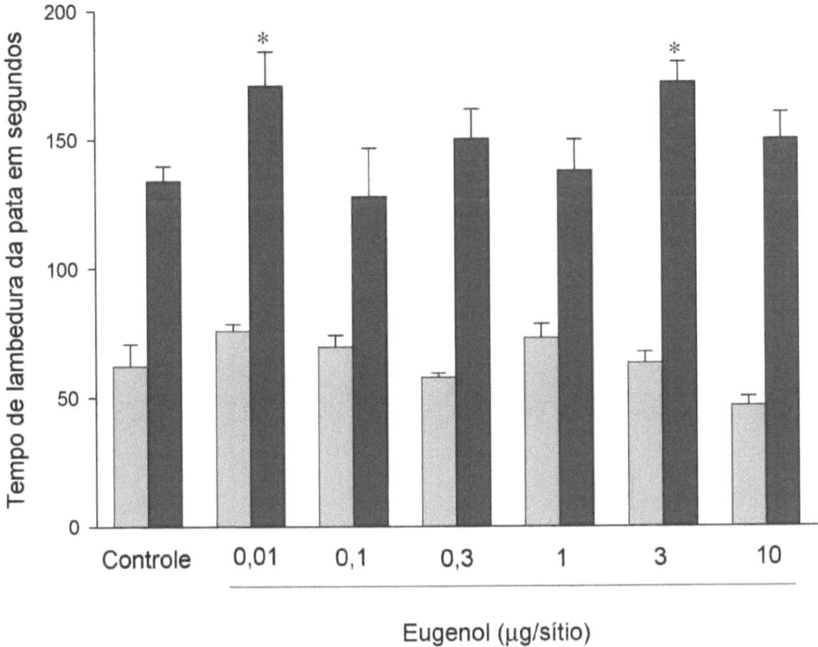

Figure 9: Evaluation of the antinociceptive effect of eugenol in the formalin test in animals pre-treated with capsazepine

(*) Statistically different from the control *p< 0.05 (ANOVA, Dunnett's test). The ordinate axis represents the time in seconds spent by the animal licking its paw and the abscissa represents the control together with each of the tested doses of eugenol. The columns represent the average licking time and the data label, at the top of each column, the standard error of the mean (SEM). n= 5 - 8 animals. Gray columns represent the first phase of the test and red columns the second phase.

Treatment	Doses (µg/sitio)	Paw licking time (seconds) 1ª PHASE ⇑	% inhibition 1st PHASE	Paw licking time (seconds) 2nd PHASE ⇑	% inhibition 2nd PHASE
Control (vehicle)	-	64,77 ± 9,24	-	128,22 ± 5,61	-
Eugenol	0,01	75,80 ± 2,81	117,03	170,80 ± 13,34**	133,21
	0,1	69,60 ± 4,36	107,46	127,80 ± 18,78	0,33
	0,3	57,80 ± 1,56	10,76	178,80 ± 16,42	139,45
	1	73,00 ± 5,44	112,71	138,00 ± 11,66	107,63
	3	63,16 ± 4,30	2,49	185,83 ± 6,90*	144,93
	10	46,83 ± 3,38	27,70	150,00 ± 10,22	116,99

Table 3 - Evaluation of the antinociceptive effect of eugenol in the formalin test in animals pre-treated with capsazepine

⇑ Values expressed as mean ± E.P.M.

*p ≤ 0.05, compared to vehicle control (ANOVA, Dunnett's test)

% inhibition with values greater than 100 mean that the dose tested increased nociception in relation to the control

n = 5 - 8 animals.

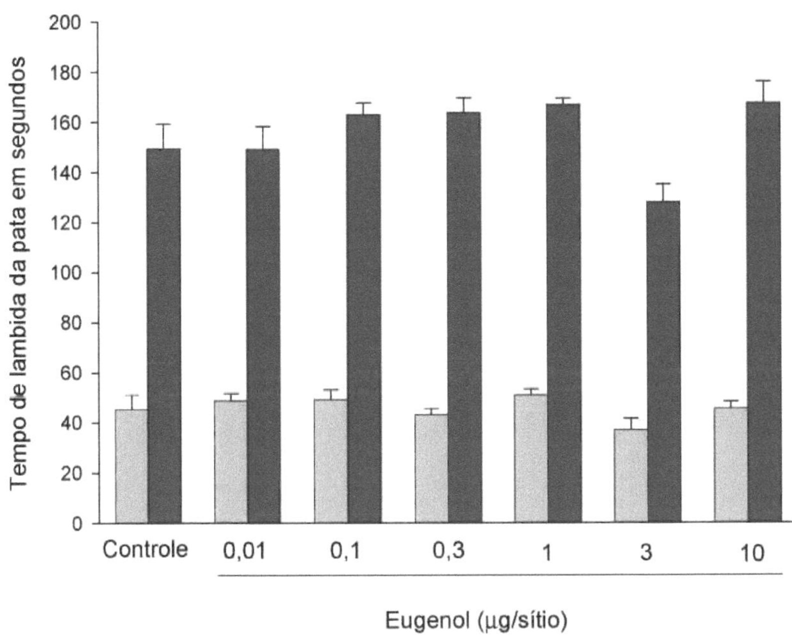

Figure 10 - Evaluation of the effect of eugenol in animals with destroyed C-fiber

(*) Statistically different from the control *p< 0.05 (ANOVA). The ordinate axis represents the time in seconds spent by the animal licking its paw and the abscissa axis represents the control together with each of the tested doses of eugenol. The columns represent the average licking time and the data label, at the top of each column, the standard error of the mean (SEM). n= 6 - 7 animals. Gray columns represent the first phase of the test and red columns the second phase.

Treatment	Doses (µg/sitio)	Paw licking time (seconds) 1ª PHASE ⇑	% inhibition 1st PHASE	Paw licking time (seconds) 2nd PHASE ⇑	% inhibition 2nd PHASE
Control (vehicle)	-	45,46 ± 5,90	-	149,46 ± 9,71	-
Eugenol	0,01	48,83 ± 2,82	107,41	149,16 ± 9,11	0,20
	0,1	49,16 ± 4,07	108,14	162,83 ± 4,78	108,95
	0,3	43,16 ± 2,41	5,06	163,50 ± 6,25	109,39
	1	51,00 ± 2,26	112,19	166,83 ± 2,57	111,62
	3	37,14 ± 4,45	18,30	112,14 ± 2,68	24,97
	10	45,50 ± 2,97	100,09	167,33 ± 8,63	111,96

Table 4 - Evaluation of the effect of eugenol in animals with destroyed C-fiber

⇑ Values expressed as mean ± E.P.M.

*$p \leq 0.05$, compared to vehicle control (ANOVA, Dunnett's test)

% inhibition with values greater than 100 mean that the dose tested increased nociception compared to the control.

n = 6 - 7 animals.

4.5. Intraplantar effect of capsaicin in the formalin test.

Capsaicin, administered intraplantarly together with formalin, caused a reduction in the nociception caused by formalin in the first phase of the test. It significantly (ANOVA, Dunnett's test) inhibited nociception at doses of 0.01; 0.1; 0.3; 1; and 10µg/sítio by 13.57 ± 3.38%, 29.63 ± 2.37%, 47.99 ± 2.12%, 48.18 ± 1.19% and 43.59 ± 3.26%, respectively. At a dose of 3µg/sitio, the inhibition was 66.54 ± 1.07% (ANOVA, Tukey test) (Figure 11, Table 5).

In the second phase of the test, capsaicin at doses of 0.3 and 10µg/sitio significantly reduced nociception (ANOVA, Dunnett's test) by 39.85 ± 1.40% and 26.33 ± 7.72%, respectively, compared to the control. At a dose of 1 µg/sitio, nociception increased by 20.68 ± 3.77% (Figure 11, Table 5).

4.6. Effect of lidocaine on formalin-induced nociception.

Lidocaine, a classic anesthetic, was administered intraplantar together with formalin. This caused a significant reduction in nociception compared to the control at all the doses tested in the first phase of the test. At doses of 0.01 (58.25 ± 3.30%); 0.1 (56.78 ± 3.15%); 1 (46.37 ± 5.01%) µg/sitio (ANOVA, Dunnett's test). At doses of 0.3 (56.59 ± 1.35%); 3 (68.97 ± 0.66%) and 10 (92.93 ± 0.51%)µg/sitio (ANOVA, Tukey Test) (Figure 12, Table 6).

In the second phase of the formalin test, lidocaine increased the nociceptive response by (24.05 ± 6.12)% at a dose of 3µg/sitio and decreased it by (29.34 ± 2.01)% at a dose of 10µg/sitio. The other doses tested had no significant effect compared to the control (Figure 12, Table 6).

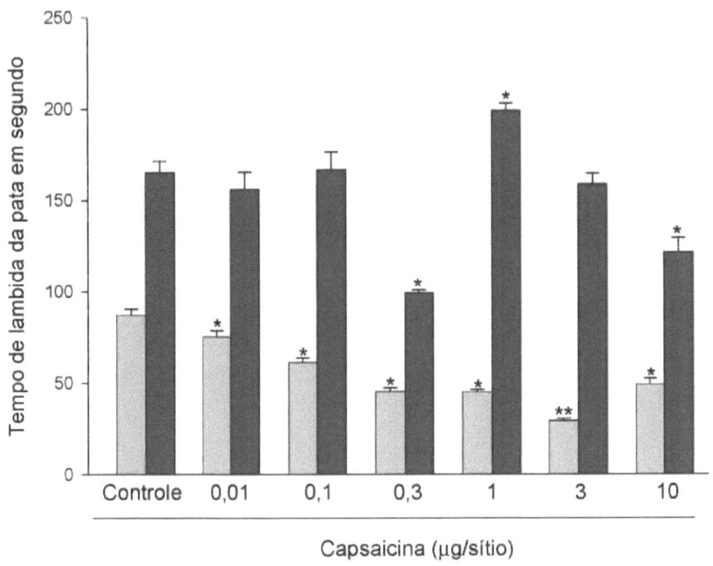

Figura 11- Intraplantar effect of capsaicin in the formalin test

(*) Statistically different from control *p < 0.05, compared to vehicle control (ANOVA, Dunnett's test); **p < 0.05, compared to vehicle control (ANOVA, Tukey test). The ordinate axis represents the time in seconds spent by the animal licking its paw and the abscissa axis represents the control together with each of the capsaicin doses tested. The columns represent the average licking time and the data label, at the top of each column, the standard error of the mean (SEM). n= 6 animals. Gray columns represent the first phase of the test and red columns the second phase.

Treatment	Doses (µg/sitio)	Paw licking time (seconds) 1ª PHASE ⇑	% inhibition 1st PHASE	Paw licking time (seconds) 2nd PHASE ⇑	% inhibition 2nd PHASE
Control (vehicle)	-	87,16 ± 3,17	-	165,16 ± 6,11	-
Capsaicin	0,01	75,33 ± 3,38 *	13,57	156,16 ± 9,21	5,45
	0,1	61,33 ± 2,37 *	29,63	166,83 ± 9,63	101,01
	0,3	45,33 ± 2,12 *	47,99	99,33 ± 1,406*	39,85
	1	45,16 ± 1,19 *	48,18	199,33 ± 3,77 *	120,68
	3	29,16 ± 1,07 **	66,54	158,66 ± 5,85	75,38
	10	49,16 ± 3,26 *	43,59	121,66 ± 7,72 *	26,33

Table 5 - Intraplantar effect of capsaicin in the formalin test

⇑ Values expressed as mean ± SEM.

*p ≤ 0.05, compared to vehicle control (ANOVA, Dunnett's test)

% inhibition with values greater than 100 mean that the dose tested increased nociception compared to the control.

n = 6 animals.

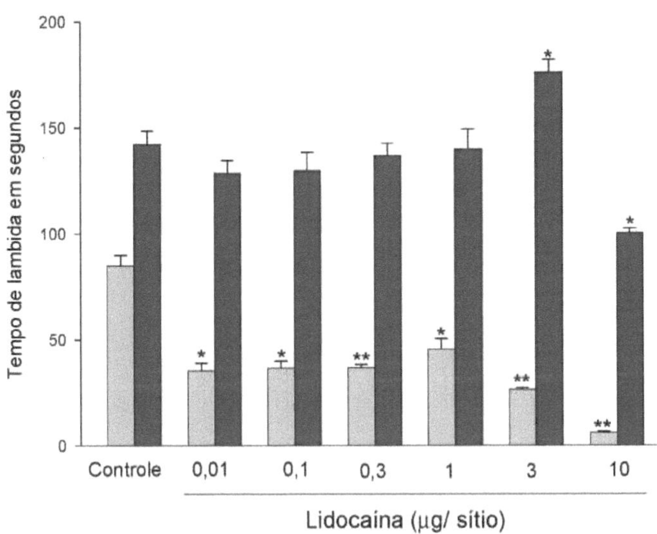

Figura 12Effect of lidocaine on formalin-induced nociception

(*) Statistically different from control *p < 0.05, compared to vehicle control (ANOVA, Dunnett's test); **p < 0.05, compared to vehicle control (ANOVA, Tukey test). The ordinate axis represents the time in seconds spent by the animal licking its paw and the abscissa represents the control together with each of the tested doses of lidocaine. The columns represent the average licking time and the data label, at the top of each column, the standard error of the mean (SEM). n= 6 - 7 animals. Gray columns represent the first phase of the test and red columns the second phase.

Treatment	Doses (µg/sitio)	Paw licking time (seconds) 1ª PHASE t	% inhibition 1st PHASE	Paw licking time (seconds) PHASE t	% inhibition 2nd 2nd PHASE
Control (vehicle)	-	84,83 ± 4,89	-	142,00 ± 6,37	-
Lidocaine	0,01	35,42 ± 3,30*	58,25	128,57 ± 6,05	9,46
	0,1	36,66 ± 3,15*	56,78	129,83 ± 8,75	8,57
	0,3	36,83 ± 1,35**	56,59	137,00 ± 5,65	3,52
	1	45,50 ± 5,01*	46,37	140,00 ± 9,40	1,41
	3	26,33 ± 0,66**	68,97	176,16 ± 6,12 *	124,05
	10	6,00 ± 0,51**	92,93	100,33 ± 2,01*	29,34

Table 6 - Effect of lidocaine on formalin-induced nociception

⇑ Values expressed as mean ± E.P.M.

% inhibition with values greater than 100 mean that the dose tested increased nociception compared to the control.

*p < 0.05, compared to vehicle control (ANOVA, Dunnett's test); **p < 0, 05, compared to vehicle control (ANOVA, Tukey test)

n = 6 - 7 animals

4.7. Comparison of the intraplantar effect of eugenol, capsaicin and lidocaine in the formalin test.

Table 7 shows the extent to which eugenol, capsaicin and lidocaine inhibited the nociception caused by intraplantar formalin. In the second phase of the test, doses with percentage values greater than 100 mean that the compound under analysis increased nociception compared to the control.

The control represents the vehicle of the solution under study.

In this table we can see that eugenol at a dose of 0.1µg/pata reduced nociception by 70.69% in the first phase. This inhibition was greater than that observed with lidocaine at the same dose. This antinociceptive effect promoted by eugenol was greater than that observed in the other doses tested.

Treatment	Doses (µg/sitio)	% inhibition 1[a] PHASE	% inhibition 2a PHASE
Eugenol	0,01	7,01	110,78*
Capsaicin		13,57*	5,44
Lidocaine		58,25*	9,45
Eugenol	0,1	**70,69***	23,81*
Capsaicin		29,63*	101,01
Lidocaine		56,78*	8,56
Eugenol	0,3	43,71*	102,10
Capsaicin		47,99*	39,85*
Lidocaine		56,59**	3,52
Eugenol	1	53,76*	104,80
Capsaicin		48,18*	120,68*
Lidocaine		46,37*	1,40
Eugenol	3	54,98*	105,40
Capsaicin		66,54**	3,93
Lidocaine		68,97**	124,05*
Eugenol	10	64,57*	102,52
Capsaicin		43,59*	26,33*
Lidocaine		92,93**	29,34*

Table 7 - Comparison of the effect of eugenol, capsaicin and lidocaine in the formalin test.

⇑ Values expressed as mean ± S.P.M. *p < 0.05, compared to vehicle control (ANOVA, Dunnett's test). **p < 0.05, compared to vehicle control (ANOVA, Tukoy's toot)

n = 6-7 animals.

5. DISCUSSION

The constituents of essential oils have been studied in order to prove their biological effects. Among these constituents, 2-methoxy-4-(2- propenyl-phenol), better known as eugenol, has been studied extensively since the last century. The great interest in studying it may be due to its various proven pharmacological effects and its low toxicity (LEAL-CARDOSO, 2002).

In this study, we deepened our knowledge of the pharmacological activities of eugenol by demonstrating its local anesthetic activity; we compared its pharmacological effect with the local effect of capsaicin and lidocaine.

We began our investigation by evaluating the effect of the local application of eugenol, since its pharmacological effects depend on its free concentration and the length of time it is exposed to the tissue (ESCOBAR, 2002), and this is also how local anesthetics are applied.

Eugenol administered intraplantar at doses of 0.01, 0.1, 0.3, 1, 3 and 10µg/sitio did not cause an increase in nociception compared to the control in the first phase of the test. However, at a dose of 30µg/sitio it caused an increase in nociception, but not significantly, and at a dose of 100µg/sitio it induced a significant increase in nociception of around 106.02%. In the second phase of the test, eugenol caused a dose-dependent increase in nociception, starting at a dose of 10µg/sitio (Figure 7, Table 1).

Since eugenol did not significantly increase nociception at doses of 0.01, 0.1, 0.3, 1, 3 and 10µg/sitio, we used these doses in the formalin test.

The formalin test has two distinct phases. The first is called neurogenic, resulting from the stimulation of peripheral nociceptors and sensory afferent fibers. The second phase of pain is associated with a peripheral inflammatory process involving the production of prostaglandins and other inflammatory mediators (SHIBATA et al, 1989; THOLSEN et al, 1992).

In this test, eugenol was able to reduce the nociception caused by formalin, in the first phase, at doses of 0.1, 0.3, 1, 3 and 10µg/sitio. The greatest antinociceptive effect was observed at a dose of 0.1 µg/sitio, which caused an inhibition of around 70.69% compared to the control (Figure 8, Table 2). This result corroborates those presented in the literature where eugenol, at low concentrations, is a reversible inhibitor of nerve activity (MARKOWITZ, 1992). This nerve inhibition is due to blocking the conduction of the action potential (OZEKI, 1975; ESCOBAR 2002).

Regarding the second phase of the test, eugenol only showed an antinociceptive effect at a dose of 0.1µg/sitio. We can suggest that in this phase the antinociceptive effect of eugenol is favored by the inhibition of prostaglandin synthesis, mainly prostaglandin E2, through the inhibition of COX-2 (ESCOBAR, 2002; KIM et al, 2003).

Bearing in mind that TRPV1 receptors are expressed in the membrane of neurons, especially those that form the small-diameter fibers sensitive to painful stimuli, i.e. the A delta fibers and the C fibers, we evaluated the effect of eugenol on these receptors through pre-treatment with capsazepine and by destroying the primary afferent fibers of the C type.

Capsazepine is a selective and competitive antagonist of type 1 vanilloid receptors. As antagonists of these receptors generally have analgesic effects, both in inflammatory and neuropathic pain, capsazepine also has these effects (CATERINA et al, 1997; OHKUBO and SHIBATA, 1997; TOMINAGA et al, 1998).

It has a significant antinociceptive effect when administered locally in both phases of formalin-induced nociception, suggesting the existence of a pro-nociceptive modulation of vanilloid receptors in peripheral tissues (GUINDON et al, 2006).

Li et al (2007) showed that pre-treatment with capsazepine decreased the effect of eugenol on voltage-activated potassium channels (VGPC), suggesting an involvement of TRPV1 receptors in the action of eugenol.

After pre-treatment with capsazepine, eugenol administered intraplantar did not reduce the nociception caused by formalin in the first phase of the test. However, in the second phase of the test, eugenol induced a significant increase in nociception at doses of 0.01 and 3µg/sitio (Figure 9, Table 3). In animals with destroyed C-fibers at birth, eugenol had no antinociceptive effect at any of the doses tested, compared to the control (Figure 10, Table 4). These data corroborate the literature, since one of the possible mechanisms by which eugenol performs its antinociceptive function is due to the interaction of eugenol with TRPV1 receptors, with an inhibition of pain transmission due to the blocking of these receptors (YANG et al, 2003).

Based on the structural similarity between the capsaicin molecule and eugenol (SZALLASI and BLUMBERG, 1999) (Figure 13) and the action of both on type 1 vanilloid receptors, we compared the local effect of eugenol with that of capsaicin in the formalin test (Table 7).

Because of this structural similarity, the two compounds must have the same molecular mechanism to produce their effects (YANG et al, 2003). Capsaicin, like eugenol, showed an antinociceptive effect in the first phase of the test. The maximum antinociceptive effect of capsaicin was observed at a dose of 3µg/sitio (66.54%) (Figure 11, Table 5). This effect is probably due to the inhibition of voltage-dependent calcium channels by both capsaicin (WU et al, 2005) and eugenol (LEE et al, 2005). The inhibition of these channels contributes to the antinociceptive effect of both eugenol and capsaicin.

It is known that the intraplantar injection of capsaicin, a substance derived from chili peppers, triggers the activation of primary afferent C fibers (amyelinated fibers, with a conduction velocity between 0.5 and 2m/s and which do not reach lamina II of the medulla) and nociceptive A delta fibers (SZALLASI & BLUMBERG, 1999). Primary afferent sensory fibers sensitive to capsaicin are important in the generation of neurogenic inflammation (HOLZER, 1988).

In the small sensory neurons of these fibers, TRPV1 receptors and their mRNAs are expressed (GUO et al, 1999). Capsaicin activates these receptors by promoting an accumulation of intracellular calcium which is important for its action (SZALLASI & BLUMBERG, 1999).

The antinociceptive properties of capsaicin have been known since the 19th century, when it was used to treat toothache. In the clinic, capsaicin is used to treat a variety of conditions, including urinary bladder hypersensitivity, neuropathic pain (such as post-herpetic neuralgia, neuropathic pain caused by diabetes, post-mastectomy pain syndrome, osteoarthritis and rheumatoid arthritis). It is also used to treat vasomotor rhinitis and paresthesia (SZALLASI AND BLUMBERG, 1999).

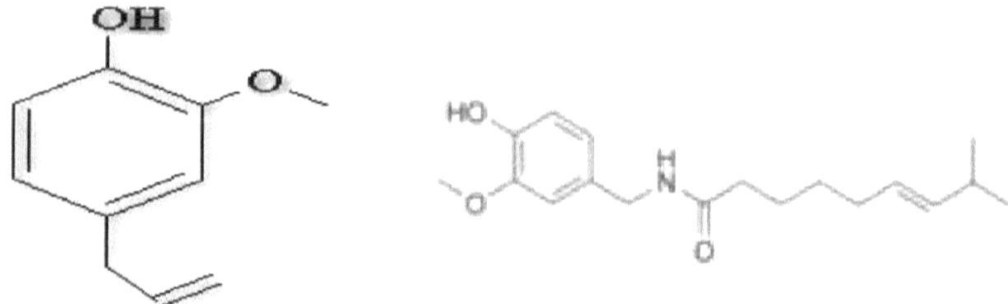

MOLECULE EUGENOL   **CAPSAICIN MOLECULE**

Figure 13: Flat structure of the Eugenol and Capsaicin molecule

Since lidocaine is the reference drug for the study of new products with anesthetic action, we compared the antinociceptive effect of eugenol with that of lidocaine in the formalin test.

Lidocaine, like eugenol, reduced the nociception caused by formalin in the first phase of the test. Its maximum antinociceptive effect was observed at a dose of 10μg/sitio (92.93%). At doses of 0.1 and 1 μg/sitio, lidocaine had an antinociceptive effect of 56.78% and 46.37%, respectively (Figure 12, Table 6). Eugenol, at these same doses, had an antinociceptive effect of 70.69% and 53.76%, respectively (Table 7). When comparing lidocaine and eugenol in this nociceptive test, it can be seen that the latter, at doses of 0.1 and 1 µg/sitio, had a greater antinociceptive effect than lidocaine.

This effect is probably due to the action of eugenol (PARK, et al, 2006) and lidocaine (FERNANDES FRACETO et al, 2005) on voltage-activated sodium channels which are important for the initiation and propagation of the action potential of excitable cells, including sensory neurons (HODGKIN AND HUXLEY, 1952).

Inhibition of voltage-activated Na^+ and Ca^{++} channels is one of eugenol's molecular mechanisms for producing antinociceptive effects (PARK et al, 2006).

Based on these results, it can be suggested that eugenol acts on TRPV1 receptors, potentially inhibiting pain transmission by blocking these receptors. Based on the data obtained, it is not possible to completely clarify that eugenol has an anesthetic effect, but it does have therapeutic relevance as an anesthetic.

The results of this study indicate that compounds obtained from natural products still have and will continue to have an important place in the process of discovering new drugs, particularly in the development of antinociceptive drugs. It is therefore suggested that future research in this area be stepped up in order to make progress in the treatment of nociception.

6. CONCLUSION

♦ Eugenol administered intraplantar does not cause an increase in nociception compared to the control at low concentrations;

♦ Eugenol has an important local antinociceptive effect at low concentrations, reducing the nociception caused by formalin;

♦ The antinociceptive effect of eugenol is due to its action on TRPV1 receptors located mainly in the C fibers;

♦ Eugenol, capsaicin and lidocaine have a local antinociceptive effect in the first phase of the formalin test.

BIBLIOGRAPHICAL REFERENCES

ABBOTT, F.V; FRANKLIN, K.B.J. **Noncompetitive antagonism of morphine analgesia by diazepam in the formalin test.** Pharmac. Bioch. and Behavior, v. 24, p.319-321, 1986.

ABRAHAM, S.K. **Anti-genotoxicity of trans-anethole and eugenol in mice.** Food Chem. Toxic., v. 39, p. 493-498, 2001.

AKOPIAN, A.N; SOUSLOVA, V; ENGLAND, S; OKUSE, K; OGATA, N; URE, J; SMITH, A; KERR, B.J; MCMAHON, S. B; BOYCE, S; et al. **The tetrodotoxinresistant sodium current SNS has a specialized function in pain pathways.** Nat. Neurosci., p. 541-548, 1999.

AL-HARBI, M. M.; QURESHI, S.; RAZA, M.; AHMED, M. M.; GIANGRECO, A. B.; SHAH, A. H. **Influence of anethole treatment on the tumor induced by Ehrlich ascites carcinoma cells in paw of Swiss albino mice.** Eur. J. Cancer Prev., v. 4(4), p. 307-18, 1995.

ALMEIDA, M.A. **Effects of eugenol on guinea pig tracheal smooth muscle.** Fortaleza, 2004. 127p. Dissertation (Master's Degree in Physiological Sciences) - Health Sciences Center, State University of Ceará.

AMONKAR, A.J.; NAGABHUSHAN, M.; D'SOUZA, A.V.; BHIDE, S.V. **Hydroxychavicol: a new phenolic antimutagen from betel leaf.** Food Chem. Toxicol., v. 24(12), p. 1321-4, 1986.

BESSON, JM. **The neurobiology of pain.** Lancet, v. 353, p. 1610-1615, 1999.

BIGHETTI, E.J.B; HIRUMA-LIMA, C.A; GRACIOSO, J.S. SOUZA BRITO, A.R.M. **Antiinflammatory and antinociceptive effects in rodents of the essential oil of Croton cajucara Benth.** J. of Pharmacy and Pharmac., v. 51, p. 1447-1453, 1999.

BUCK, S.H.; BURKS, T.F. **Capsaicin: hot new pharmacological tool.** Trends in Pharmac. Sci., v.4, p. 84-87, 1983.

BUDAVARI, S. **The merck index. Merck & Co. Inc.**, Rahway, N.J., 1996.

BOUTHILLIER L.; CHARBONNEAU M.; BRODEUR J. **Assessment of the role of glutathione conjugation in the protection afforded by anethol dithiolthione against hexachloro-I,3-butadiene-induced nephrotoxicity.** Toxicol. Appl. Pharmac., v.139 (1), p. 177-85, 1996.

BROWN EM. **Extracellular Ca^{+2} sensing, regulation of parathyroid cell function, and role of Ca^{+2} and other ions as extracellular (first) messengers.** Physiol. Rev., p. 371-

411, 1991.

CATERINA, M.J., JULIUS, D. **The vanilloid receptor: a molecular gateway to the pain pathway.** Annu. Rev. Neurosci., v.24, p.487 and 517, 2001.

CATERINA, M.J., SCHUMACHER, M.A., TOMINAGA, M., ROSEN, T.A., LEVINE, J.D., JULIUS, D. **The capsaicin receptor: a heat-activated ion channel in the pain pathway.** Nature, v.389, p.816-824. 1997.

CORREL, C.C; PHELPS, P.T; ANTHES, J.C; UMLAND, S; GREENFEDER, S. **Cloning and pharmacological characterization of mouse** TRPv1. Neurosc. Lett., v. 370, p.55-60, 2004.

COSTA, P.R.R. **Safrole and eugenol: study of chemical reactivity and use in the synthesis of biologically active natural products and their derivatives.** Quimica Nova, v. 23, n. 3, p. 357-369, 2000.

CUNHA, M. A; COPATTI, C. E; GARCIA, L. O; FONSECA, M. B; FERREIRA, F.W; MALDANER, G; MOREL, A. F; LORO, V. L; BALDISSEROTTO, B. **Cortisol levels in jundiâs (*Rhamdia Quelen*) exposed to clove oil (*Eugenol*) and *Condalia Buxifolia* extract.** Quaciência Bento Gonçalves. Proceedings, 2006.

CRAVEIRO, A.C, FERNANDES, A.G; ANDRADE, C.H.S; MATOS, F.J.A; ALENCAR, J.W; MACHADO, M.I.L. **Óleos essenciais de plantas do Nordeste.** Edições UFC, Fortaleza, Ce, 1981.

DALLMEIR, K; CARLINI, E. A. **Anesthetic, hypothermic, myorelaxant and anticonvulsant effects of synthetic Eugenol derivates.** Pharmac., v.22, p.113127, 1981.

DAVIS, J.B; GRAY, J; GUNTHORPE, M.J; HATCHER, J.P; DAVEY, P.T; OVEREND, P; HARRIES, M.H; LATCHAM, J; CLAPHAM, C; ATKINSON, K; HUGHES, S.A; RANCE, K., GRAU, E; HARPER, A.J; PUGH, P.L; ROGERS, D.C; BINGHAM, S; RANDALL, A; SHEARDOWN, S.A. **Vanilloid receptor-1 is essential for inflammatory thermal hyperalgesia.** Nature, v.405, p.183-187, 2000.

DERAEDT, R; JOUGNEY, S; DELEVALCEE, F; FALHOUT, M. **Release of prostaglandins E and F in algogenic reaction and its inhibition.** Eur. J. of Pharmac., v. 61, p. 17-24, 1980.

DIP, E.C; PEREIRA, N.A; FERNANDES, P.D.C. **Ability of eugenol to reduce tongue edema induced by *Dieffenbachia picta* Schott in mice.** Toxic., v. 43, p. 729-735, 2004.

DRUKARCH, B.; SCHEPENS, E.; STOOF, J. C.; LANGEVELD, C. H. **Anethole dithiolethione prevents oxidative damage in glutathione-depleted astrocytes.** Eur. J.

Pharmacol., v. 25; 329(2-3), p. 259-62, 1997.

ESCOBAR, R. G. **Eugenol: Pharmacological and toxicological properties. Advantages and disadvantages of its use.** Ver Cubana Estomatol, v. 39, 2002.

FENG, J; LIPTON, J. M. **Eugenol: antipyretic activity in rabbits.** Neuropharmac., v.26 no 12, p.1775-1778, 1987.

FERNANDES FRACETO, L; SPISNI, A; SCHREIER, S; de PAULA, E. **Differential effects of uncharged aminoamide local anesthetics on phospholipid bilayers, as montored by 1H-NMR measurements.** Biophys. Chem., v. 115, p. 11-18, 2005.

FRANCIS, A. R.; SHETTY, T. K.; BHATTACHARYA, R. K. **Modification of the mutagenicity of aflatoxin B1 and N-methyl-N'-nitro-N-nitrosoguanidine by certain phenolic compounds.** Cancer. Lett., v. 45(3), p. 177-82, 1989.

FÜRST, S. **Transmitters involved in antinociception in the spinal cord.** Brain Res. Bull, v.48; p.129-141, 1999.

GEPPETTI,P; TREVISANI, M. **Activation and sensitization of the vanilloid receptor: role in gastrointestinal inflammation and function.** Br. J. Pharmacol., v. 141, p. 127-132, 2004.

GUINDON, J; VERME, J.L; LÉAN, A.D.; Piomelli, D; Beaulieu, P. **Synergistic antinociceptive effects of anandamide, an endocannabinoid, and nonsteroidal anti-inflammatory drugs in peripheral tissue: A role for endogenous fatty-acid ethanolamides?** Eur. J. of Pharmac., v. 550, p. 68-77, 2006.

GUO, A; VULCHANOVA, L; WANG, J; LI, X; ELDE, R. **Immunocytochemical localization of the vanilloid receptor 1 (VR1): relationship to neuropeptides, the P2X3 purinoceptor and IB4 binding sites.** Eur. J. Neurosci., v. 11, p. 946 and 958, 1999.

GYIRES, K; TORMA, Z. **The use of the writhing test in mice for screening different types of analgesics.** Arch. Int. Pharmacodyn. Ther, v. 267, p. 131-140, 1984.

HAAS, D. **An update on local anesthetics in dentistry.** J. of the Canadian Dental Ass., v. 68, numbor 9, 2002.

HARDIE, R.C; MINKE B. **Novel Ca^{++} channels underlying transduction in Drosophila photoreceptors: implications for phosphoinositidemediated Ca^{+2} mobilization, Trends.** Neurosci., v. 16, p. 371-376, 1993.

HODGKIN, A.L; HUXLEY, A.F. **A quantitative description of membrane current and its application to conduction and excitation in nerve.** J. Physiol., v. 117, p. 500-544, 1952.

HOLZER, P. **Capsaicin: cellular target, mechanisms of action, and selectivity for yhin sensory neurons.** Pharmacol. Rev., v. 43(2), p. 143-201, 1991.

HOLZER, P. **Local effector functions of capsaicin-sensitive sensory nerve endings: involvement of tachykinins, calcitonin gene-related peptide and other neuropeptides.** Neurosc., v.24, p. 739-768, 1988.

HUME, W. R. **Effect of eugenol on constrictor responses in blood vessels of the rabbit ear.** J. Dent. Res., v. 62(9), p. 1013-5, 1983.

HUNSKAAR, S; HOLE, K. **Formalin test in mice a useful technique for evaluating mild analgesics.** J. Neurosci. Meth., v. 14, p. 69-76, 1985.

HUNSKAAR, S; HOLE, K. **The formalin test in mice: dissociation between inflammatory and non-inflammatory pain.** Pain, v. 30, p. 103-114, 1987.

HUNSKAAR, S; HOLE, K; ROSLAND, H. **Modification of the antinociceptive effect of morphine by diazepam.** Pain, v.30, p.S43, 1987.

IKEDA, Y; UENO, A; NARABA, H; OH-ISHI, S. **Involvement of vanilloid receptor VR1 and prostanoids in the acid- induced writhing responses of mice.** Life Sci., v. 69, p. 2911-2919, 2001.

INOUE, L.A.K.A; SANTOS NETO, C; MORAES, G. **Clove oil as anaesthetic for juveniles of matrinxa Brycon cephalus (Gunther, 1869).** Ciência Rural, Santa Maria, v.33, n.5, p.943- 947, 2003.

ITO, M; MURAKAMI, K; YOSHINO, M. **Antioxidant action of eugenol compounds: role of metal ion in the inhibition of lipid peroxidation.** Food and Chem. Toxic., v. 43, p. 461-466, 2005.

JOOHYENG, L.; VICENZO, Di Marzo; JONATHAN, M.B. **A role for vanilloid receptor 1(TRPV1) and endocannabinnoid signaling in the regulation of spontaneous and L-DOPA induced locomotion in normal and resespine-treated rats.** Neuropharmacol., v.51, p. 557-565, 2006.

KIM, S.S; OH, O.J; MIN, H.Y; PARK, E.J; KIM, Y; PARK, H.J; NAMHAN, Y; LEE, S.K. **Eugenol suppresses cyclooxygenase-2 expression in lipopolysaccharide-stimulated mouse macrophage RAW264.7 cells.** Life Sci., v.73, p. 337- 48, 2003.

KIM, H. M; LEE, E. H; KIM, C. Y; CHUNG, J. G; KIM, S. H; LIM, J.P; SHIN, T. Y. **Antianaphylactic properties of eugenol.** Pharmac. Research, v 48, p. 3620-3632, 1997.

KOTHARI, S.K; BHATTACHRYA, A.K; RAMESH. S. **Essential oil yield quality of methyl** eugenol rich *Ocimum tenuiflorum* L.f. (syn. *O. sanctum L.*) grown in south India as influnced by method of harvest. J of Chromat A, v. 1054, p. 67-72, 2004.

KUMARAVELU, P; SUBRAMANLYAM, S; DAKSHINAMOORTHY, D. P; DEVARAF, N. S. **The antioxidant effect of eugenol on CCL4 -induced erytrocyte damage in rats.** J. Nutr. Biochem., v. 7, p. 23-28, 1996.

KWAK, J.Y; JUNG, J.Y; HWANG, S.W; LEE, W.T., OH, U. **A capsaicin receptor antagonist, capsazepine, reduces inflammation-induced hyperalgesic responses in the rat: evidence for an endogenous capsaicin-like substance.** Neurosc., v.86, p. 619-626, 1998.

LAHLOU, S; CALDAS MAGALHAES, P.J; LEAL-CARDOSO, J.H; DUARTE, G.P. **Cardiovascular Effects of Eugenol, a Phenolic Compound Present in Many Plant Essential Oils, in Normotensive Rats.** J. of Cardiov. Pharmac., v. 43(2) p. 250-257, 2004.

LAURETTI, G.R. **Mechanisms involved in the analgesia of intravenous lidocaine.** Rev. Bras. de Anestesiol., v.58, 2008.

LAWSON, S.N. **Phenotype and function of somatic primary afferent nociceptive neurones with C-, Adelta- or Aalpha/beta-fibres.** Exp. Physiol., v.87, p. 239-244, 2002.

LEAL-CARDOSO, J.H; MOREIRA, M.R; PINTO DA CRUZ, G.M; MORAIS, S.M; LAHLOU, M.S; COELHO-DE-SOUZA, A.N. **Effects of essential oil of alpinia zerumbet on the compound action potential of the rat sciatic nerve.** Phytomed., v. 11, p. 549-553, 2003.

LEAL-CARDOSO, J.H; LAHLOU, S; COELHO-DE-SOUZA, A.N; CRIDDLE, D.N.; PINTO DUARTE, G.I; SANTOS, M.A; MAGALHAES, P.J. **Inhibitory actions of eugenol on rat isolated ileum.** Can. J. Physiol. Pharmacol., v. 80, p. 901-6, 2002.

LEAL-CARDOSO, J.H; COELHO-DE-SOUZA, A.N; SOUZA, I.T; FIGUEIREDO, I.M. **Effects of eugenol on excitation-contraction coupling in skeletal muscle.** Arch. Int. Pharmacodyn. Ther., v. 327, p. 113-24, 1994.

LEE, J; DI MARZO, V; BROTCHIE, J.M. **A role for vanilloid receptor 1 (TRPV1) and endocannabinnoid signaling in the regulation of spontaneous and L- DOPA induced locomotion in normal and reserpine treated rates.** Neuropharmacol., v. 51, p. 557-565, 2006.

LEE, M.H; YEON, K.Y; PARK, C.K; LI, H.Y; FANG, Z; KIM, M.S; CHOI, S.Y; LEE, S.J; LEE, S; PARK, K; LEE, J.H; KIM, J.S; OH, S.B. **Eugenol inhibits calcium currents in dental afferent neurons.** J. Dent. Res., v. 84, p. 848-851, 2005.

LI, H.Y; PARK. C.K; KIM, J.S; OH, S.B. **Eugenol inhibits voltage-gated potassium currents in trigeminal ganglion neurons.** Eur. J. of Pain, v. 11, p. 158, 2007.

MADEIRA, S.V.F; RABELO, M; SOARES, P.M.G; SOUZA, E.P; MEIRELES, A.V.P; MONTENEGRO, C; LIMA, R.F; ASSREUY, A.M.S; CRIDDLE, D.N. **Temporal variation of chemical composition and relaxant action of the essential oil of *Ocimum gratissimum* L. (Labiatae) on guinea-pig ileum.** Phytomed., v. 12, p.506509, 2005.

MALAMED, S. F. **Manual of local anesthesia.** 3ª edition Guanabara Koogan, 1993.

MANSUY, D; SASSI, A; DANSETTE, P. M; PLAT, M. **A new potent inhibitor of lipid peroxidation in vitro and *in vivo*, the hepatoprotective drug anisyldithiolyhione.** Biochem. Biophys. Res Commun., v. 28, 135(3), p. 1015-21, 1986.

MARKOWITZ, K; MOYNIHAN, M; LIU, M; KIM, S. **Biologic properties of eugenol and zinc oxide-eugenol. A clinically oriented review.** Oral Surg. Oral Med. Oral Pathol., v. 73(6), p. 729-37, 1992.

MATOS, M.J.A; FERNANDES, A. **Reports of excursions of the program chemical study of essential oils of native and cultivated plants in the northeast.** BNB-CNPq-UFC agreements, 1975-1978. Mimeographed.

MERSKEY, H; BOGDUK, N. **Classification of chronic pain: description of chronic pain syndromes and definitions of pain terms.** IASP Press: Seatte, 1994.

MILLAN, M.J. **The induction of pain: an integrative review.** Prog. Neurobiol., v. 57, p. 1-164, 1999.

MONTELL K; RUBIN G.M. **Molecular characterization of the Drosophila trp locus: a putative integral membrane protein required for phototransduction.** Neurone, v. 2, p.1313-1323, 1989.

MORRISON, R; BOYD, R. **Organic Chemistry.** Allyn and Bacon, Inc., Boston, 1961.

NAGABABU, E; LAKSHMAIAH, N. **Inhibition of microsomal lipid peroxidation and monooxygenase activities by eugenol.** Free Radic. Res., v. 20, p. 253-66, 1994.

NAIDU, K.A. **Eugenol - an Inhibitor of Lipoxygenase-Dependent Lipid Peroxidation. Prostaglandins Leukotr.** Essent Fatty Acids, v. 53, p. 381-383, 1995.

NELSON, E.K. **The constitution of capsaicin-the pungent principle of capsicum.** J. Am. Chem. Soc., v.41, p.1115-1117, 1919.

NISHIJIMA, H; UCHIDA, R; KAMEYAMA, K; KAWAKAMI, N; OHKUBO, T; KITAMURA, K.

Mechanisms mediating the vasorelaxing ation of eugenol, a pungent oil, on rabbit arterial tissue. Jpn. J. Pharmacol., v. 79, p. 327-334, 1999.

OGATA, N; OHISHI, Y. **Molecular diversity of structure and function of the voltage-gated Na⁺ channels.** Jpn. J Pharmacol., v. 88, p. 365-377, 2002.

OHKUBO, Y, SHIBATA, M. **The selective capsaicin antagonist capsazepine abolishes the antinociceptive action of eugenol and guaicol.** J. Dent. Res., v.76, p.848-851, 1997.

OZEKI, M. **The effects of eugenol on the nerve and muscle in cryfish.** Comp. Biochem. Physiol., v. 50, p. 183-191, 1975.

PARK, C.K; LI, H.Y; YEON, K.Y; JUMG, S.J; CHOI, S.Y; LEE, S.J; LEE, S; PARK, K; KIM, J.S; OH, S.B. **Eugenol inhibits sodium currents in dental afferent neurons.** J. Dent. Res., v. 85, p. 900-904, 2006.

PATEL, M; SAMSOON, G; SWAMI, A; MORGAN B. **Posture and spread of hyperbaric bupivacaine in parturients using combined spinal epidural technique.** Can. J. Anaesth., v. 40(10), p. 943-946, 1993.

PESSOA, L.M; MORAIS, S.M; BEVILAQUA, C.M.L; LUCIANO, J.H.S. **Anthelmintic activity of essential oil of *Ocimum gratissimum* Linn. And Eugenol against *Haemonchus contortus*.** Veterin. Parasit., v. 109, p. 59-63, 2002.

Probem Laboratório de Produtos farmacêuticos e Odontológicos S/A.

www.dentsply.com.br Registered with ANVISA/MS 1.0993.0002.001-1.

RAGHAVENRA, H; DIWAKR, B.T; LOKESH, B.R.; NAIDU, K.A. **Eugenol-the active principle from cloves inhibits 5-lipoxygenase activity and leukotriene-C4 in human PMNL cells.** Prostag. Leukot. Essent. Fatty Acids, v.74, p.23-7, 2006.

RASMUSSEN, H. **Cellular calcium metabolism.** Ann. Intern. Med., v. 98, p. 809816, 1983.

REDDY, B. S. **Chemoprevention of colon cancer by dietary administration of naturally-occurring and related synthetic agents.** Adv. Exp. Med. Biol., v. 400B, p.931-6, review, 1997.

REDDY, B. S. **Chemoprevention of colon cancer by minor dietary constituents and their synthetic analogues.** Prev. Med., v.25 (1), p. 48-50. Review, 1996.

REDDY, A.C; LOKESH, B.R. **Studies on anti-inflammatory activity of spice principles and dietary n-3 polyunsaturated fatty acids on carrageenan-induced inflammation in rats.** Ann. Nutr. Metab., v. 38, p. 349-358, 1994.

REDDY, B. S; RAO, C. V; RIVENSON, A; KELLOFF, G. **Chemoprevention of colon carcinogenesis by organosulfur compounds.** Cancer Res., v 1; 53(15), p.3493-8, 1993.

ROCHA, A.P.C; LEMONICA, L; BARROS, G.A.M. **Uso de medicações por via subaracnóide no Tratamento da dor crônica.** Rev. Bras. de Anestesiol. v.52, p.628-643, 2002.

ROMPELBERG, C. J; PLOEMEN, J. H; JESPERSE, S; VAN DER GREEF, J.; VERHAGEN, H; VAN BLADEREN, P. J. **Inhibition of rat, mouse and human glutathione S-transferase by eugenol and its oxidation products.** Chem. Biol. Interact, v. 5, 99(1-3), p. 85-97, 1996.

ROOD, J.P. **Some anatomical and physiological causes of failure to achieve mandibular analgesia.** Brit. J. Oral Surg., v. 15, p.75, 1977/1978.

ROSS, L.G; ROSS, B. **Anaesthetic and sedative techniques for aquatic animals.** 2ed. Oxford: Blackwell Sci., 1999.

ROUBACH, R; GOMES, L.C; FONSECA, F.A.L; VAL, A.L. **Eugenol as an efficacious anaesthetic for tambaqui, _Colossoma macropomum_ (Cuvier).** Aquaculture Res. v.36, n.11, p.1056 - 1061,2005.

ROUBACH, R; GOMES, L.C. **The use of anesthetics during fish handling.** Panor. da Aqüic., v.66, n.2, 2001.

RUSSO, C.M., BROSE, W.G. **Chronic pain.** Ann. Rev. Med. v. 49, p. 123-133, 1998.

SAITOH, C; KITADA, C; UCHIDA, W; CHANCELLOR, M.B; GROAT, W.C; YOSHIMURA, N. **The differential contractile responses to capsaicin and anandamide in muscle strips isolated from the rat urinary bladder.** Eur. J. of Pharmac., v. 570, p. 182-187, 2007.

SENANAYAKE, U.M; WILLS, B.H; Lee, T.H. **Biosynthesis of eugenol and cinnamic aldehyde in _Cinnamomum zeylanicum._** Phytoch., v.16, p-2032-2033, 1977.

SHARMA, J.N; SRIVASTAVA, K.C; GAN, E.K. **Suppressive effects of eugenol and ginger oil on arthritic rats.** Pharmac., v. 49, p.314-318, 1994.

SHIBATA, M; OHKUBO, T; TAKAHASHI, H; INOKI, R. **Modified formalin test: characteristic biphasic pain response.** Pain, v. 38, p. 347-352, 1989.

SIEBEN, S; HERTL, M; MASAOUDI, T. A; MERK, H. F; BLOMEKE, **B. Characterization of T cell responses to fragrances.** Toxicol. Appl. Pharmacol., v. 172, p. 172-178, 2001.

SIEMONEIT, K. D; ZIPF, H. F; DITTMANN E. C. **Unter such ungen zur endoanasthetischen und hypnotisch narkotischen wirkung von 2-methoxy-4- allyl-**

phenoxyessigsaure-N,N-diathylamid und verwandten phenolderivaten. Arch. Int. Pharmacodyn., v.164, p. 30-46, 1966.

SIMOES, C.M.O; SCHENKEL, E.P; MELLO, J.C.P. **Farmacognosia da planta ao medicamento.** Porto Alegre, Ed. da Universidade UFRGS, 1999.

SMALL, C.B. **Anesthetic efficacy of metomidate and comparison of plasma cortisol responses to tricaine methanesulphonate, quinaldine and clove oil anesthetized channel catfish Ictalurus punctatus.** Aquac., v. 218, p. 177-185, 2003.

SOUZA, T.F.S.N.N. de **Antinociceptive and anti-edematogenic effect of eugenol.** Fortaleza, 2007. Dissertation (Master's Degree in Physiological Sciences) - Health Sciences Center, State University of Ceará.

SZALLASI, A., BLUMBERG, P.M. **Vanilloid (capsaicin) receptors and mechanisms.** Pharm. Rev., v.51, p.159-212, 1999.

SMITH, K.A. **Interleukin-2: inception, impact, and implications.** Sci, v. 240, p. 1169-1176, 1988.

SOUZA, J.L.C. **Effect of eugenol on voltage-dependent Na channels$^+$** . Fortaleza, 2005. 106p. Dissertation (Master's Degree in Physiological Sciences) - Health Sciences Center, State University of Ceará.

SOUZA-JUNIOR, V.B; ALVES-JUNIOR, T.T. **The effectiveness of clove oil (eugenol) as an anesthetic in the handling of juvenile sea bass *Centropomus undecimalis*, kept in captivity.** Aquaciência, Bento Gonçalves Anais, 2006.

STOHS, S. J; LAWSON, T. A; ANDERSON, L; BUEDING, E. **Effects of oltipraz, BHA, ADT and cabbage on glutathione metabolism, DNA damage and lipid peroxidation in old mice.** Mech. Agein Dev., v. 37(2), p. 137-45, 1986.

TAIRA, J; IKEMOTO, T; YONEYA, T; HAGI, A; MURAKAMI, A; MAKINO, K. **Essential oil phenyl propanoids. Useful as OH scavengers?** Free Radic. Res. Commun., v. 16, p. 197-204, 1992.

TJølsen A; BERGE O.G; HUNSKAAR, S; ROSLAND, J. H; HOLE, K. **The formalin test: an evaluation of the method.** Pain, v.51 5-17, 1992.

TOMINAGA, M; CATERINA, M.J; MALMBERG, A.B; ROSEN, T.A; GILBERT, H; SKINNER, K; RAUMANN, B.E; BASBAUM, A.I; JULIUS, D. **The cloned capsaicin receptor integrates multiple pain-producing stimuli.** Neuronsc., v.21, p.531-543, 1998.

UEDA- NAKAMURA, T; MENDONÇA-FILHO, R.R; MORGADO-DiAZ, J.A; MAZA, P.K; FILHO, B.P.D; CORTEZ, D.A.G; ALVINO, D.S; ROSA, M. do S.S; LOPES, A.H.C.S; ALVIANO, C.S; NAKAMURA, C.V. **Antileishmanial activity of Eugenol- rich essential oil from *Ocimum gratissimum.*** Parasit. Int., v. 55, p. 99-105, 2006.

USTA, J; KREYDIYYEH, S; BAJAKIAN, K; NAKKASH-CHMAISSE, H. **In vitro effect of eugenol and cinnamaldehyde on membrane potential and respiratory chain complexes in isolated rat liver mitochondria.** Food and Chemical. Toxic., v. 40, p.935-940, 2002.

VIDAL, L.V.O; FURUYA, W.M; GRACIANO, T.S; SCHAMBER, C.R; SILVA, L.C.R; SANTOS,L.D; SOUZA, S.R. **Eugenol as anaesthetic for matrinxa juveniles *("Brycon cephalus".*** Rev. Bras. Saùde Prod. An., v.8, n.4, p. 335-342, 2007.

VIDAL, L. V. O; ALBINATI, R.C.B; ALBINATI, A.C.L; MACÊDO, G.R. de. **Use of Eugenol as an Anesthetic for the Management of Juvenile Pintado (*Pseudoplatystoma corruscans*).** Acta Scientiarum Biol. Sci., Maringà, v.28, n. 3, 2006.

YAMAMOTO, Y.; TAGA, K; YOSHIDA, T; KAMAGA, H; VEDA, I. **Temperature dependence of thermodynamic activity in volatile anesthetics: Correlation between anesthetic potency and activity.** J. of Colloid and Interface Sci., v. 301, p. 488-492, 2006.

YANG, B.H; PIAO, Z.G; KIM, Y.B; LEE, C.H; PARK, K; KIM, J.S; OH, S.B. **Activation of vanilloid receptor 1 (VR$_1$) by eugenol.** J. Dent. Res., v.82, p.781785, 2003.

ZIMMERMANN, M. **Ethical guidelines for investigations of experimental pain in conscious animals.** Pain. v.16, p. 109-110, 1983.

WU, Z.Z; CHEN, S .R; PAN, H.L. **Transient receptor potential vanilloid type 1 activation down-regulates voltage-gated calcium channels through calciumdependent calcineurin in sensory neurons.** J. Biol. Chem., v. 280, p. 1814218151, 2005.

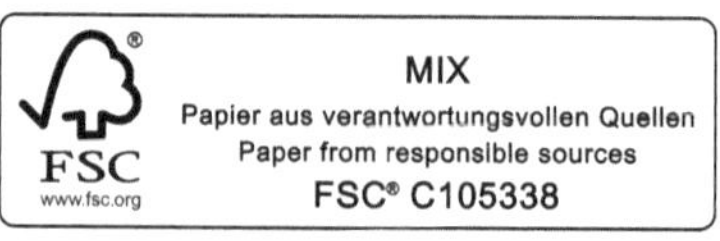

Printed by Books on Demand GmbH, Norderstedt / Germany